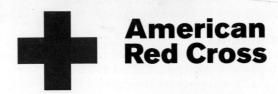
American
Red Cross

FIRST AID
AND SAFETY
FOR BABIES
AND CHILDREN

StayWell®

A MediMedia USA Company

Dedication

This book and DVD set is dedicated to parents and soon-to-be parents who, on a daily basis, are responsible for the day-to-day health and safety of their children.

Acknowledgments

This *First Aid and Safety for Babies and Children* book and DVD set was developed and produced through the combined efforts of the American Red Cross and StayWell. Without the commitment to excellence of both employees and volunteers, this product could not have been created.

Note to Our Readers

The information contained in this book and on the enclosed DVD is not intended as a substitute for training and materials you would receive in a Red Cross First Aid and CPR/AED class. We urge you to call your local Red Cross chapter to schedule training soon.

When you see this DVD icon in the book margins ⊚, it means the skill is demonstrated or the topic is covered in greater detail on the enclosed DVD.

The editors agreed that to avoid awkward and wordy "he or she" and "him or her" sentence constructions, we alternated the gender reference throughout the text when referring to a child or infant. Similarly, to avoid awkward and wordy "an infant and a child" and "infants and children" sentence constructions, use of the term "child" or "children" generally refers to both infants and children.

Printed in China.
StayWell
780 Township Line Rd.
Yardley, PA 19067

Library of Congress Cataloging-in-Publication Data

First aid and safety for babies and children.
        p. cm. — (Be Red Cross ready safety series ; vol. 5)
    ISBN 978-1-58480-413-0
    1. Pediatric emergencies—Popular works. 2. First aid in illness and injury—Popular works. I. American Red Cross.
    RJ370.F574 2009
    618.92'0025—dc22

                                        2008033586

ISBN: 978-1-58480-413-0

09 10 11 12/9 8 7 6 5 4 3 2 1

About the American Red Cross

Mission of the American Red Cross
The American Red Cross, a humanitarian organization led by volunteers and guided by its Congressional Charter and the Fundamental Principles of the International Red Cross Movement, will provide relief to victims of disaster and help people prevent, prepare for and respond to emergencies.

The American Red Cross helps people prevent, prepare for and respond to emergencies. Last year, almost a million volunteers and 35,000 employees helped victims of almost 75,000 disasters; taught lifesaving skills to millions; and helped U.S. service members separated from their families stay connected. Almost 4 million people gave blood through the Red Cross, the largest supplier of blood and blood products in the United States. The American Red Cross is part of the International Red Cross and Red Crescent Movement. An average of 91 cents of every dollar the Red Cross spends is invested in humanitarian services and programs. The Red Cross is not a government agency; it relies on donations of time, money and blood to do its work.

Fundamental Principles of the International Red Cross and Red Crescent Movement

Humanity

Impartiality

Neutrality

Independence

Voluntary Service

Unity

Universality

Table of Contents

Foreword

As a parent, you know that nothing is more important than keeping your children safe and secure. We know that, too. For more than 125 years, the American Red Cross has helped parents like you protect your children at home and in the community, whether on a daily basis or when emergencies occur.

Your purchase of this book and DVD set is one of the most important steps you can take to keep that commitment. Because the most fundamental aspect of keeping your children healthy is prevention, the first part of this book addresses what you can do to prevent emergencies. And if, despite your best efforts, an accident or other emergency occurs, then this book will help you be prepared to know what to do.

Emergency preparedness begins in your own home. Having the supplies you need, the skills to use them and a plan in advance helps ensure your family can cope not only with private family emergencies but also with large-scale regional disasters, like hurricanes.

Throughout this book there are recommendations for improving your environment and preparing for emergencies that you and your children (depending on their age) can work on together. For instance, involve your school-age child in creating a first aid and disaster supplies kit. Show your preschooler why you are tying up curtain cords, and get him or her to help you make sure you have taken care of all the cords in the house.

Read through the first aid section and watch the DVD together, so you will all know what to do if any one of you needs help.

Although the information contained within this manual is a good start, we encourage you to take the next step and sign up for a first aid and CPR/AED training course at your local Red Cross chapter. You are now on the path to giving yourself and your family the gift of being Red Cross Ready.

Best wishes for a safe, secure future,

David Markenson, MD, FAAP
Chief, Pediatric Emergency Medicine
Maria Fareri Children's Hospital
Westchester Medical Center

Associate Professor of Pediatrics and Public Health
New York Medical College

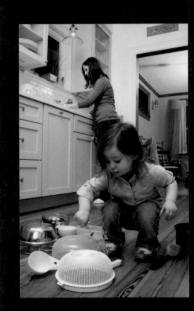

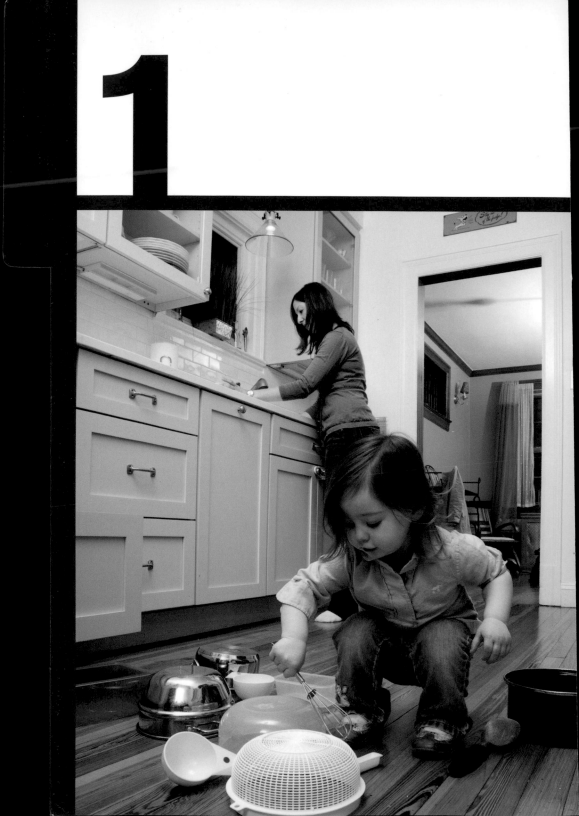

1

Keeping Your Child Safe

Your home should be a safe place for your children, the safest place outside of your arms. By taking a careful look around your home with your child's safety in mind, you can spot potential hazards and remove them before anything happens. In this chapter, you will learn what steps to take to reduce the risk of accidents and keep your children safe and healthy.

Safety In and Around the Home

Accidents are the leading cause of injury and death in children. While certain things, such as the weather, are outside of your control, there is much you can do to create a safer environment for your children, beginning in your own home. For instance, that cord hanging from the window blind in the living room? Shorten it or remove it altogether so young children can't become tangled in it and suffocate. Those perfumes on your dresser? They look so pretty a preschooler might decide to drink them, risking poisoning, so put them away where your children can't find them. And teach your children to walk, not run, through your home; otherwise, your energetic first grader might trip and fall into the corner of the slate coffee table, suffering a serious head or eye injury. The next few pages provide a room-by-room guide to help you make your home a safer place for your children.

Halls and Stairs

Halls and stairs are ideal places for trips and falls. To prevent them:

- Keep stairs clear of toys and other objects.
- Make sure staircases are well lit.
- Always use safety gates at the top and bottom of staircases until your children have learned how to walk, and go up and down the stairs and understand safety around stairs. Do not use pressure-mounted safety gates at the top of staircases; use only wall-mounted safety gates in these areas.
- Consider carpeting wood stairs or installing nonslip treads to prevent slips.
- Equip all stairs with sturdy handrails and teach your children to use the railing.

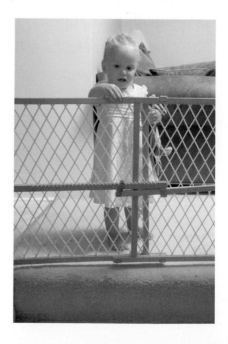

- Don't let your children slide down banisters.
- Install protective barriers on balconies to prevent children from slipping through the bars.

Doors. You might not think a door can be a safety hazard, but a child's finger can become caught and severed in a suddenly slamming door. Meanwhile, open access to rooms like kitchens and baths can create a tempting, yet dangerous opportunity for curious babies and toddlers. To safety-proof your doors:

- Install slow-closing hinges so doors close gently.
- When practical, use safety devices that prevent doors from being completely closed.
- Remove locks from doors so children can't become locked inside a room, or make sure you have a key to all doors with locks.
- Install gates in doorways to block access to rooms, like the kitchen or bathroom, which may be unsafe for a crawling baby or young child.

Floors. Your floors are a superhighway for crawling babies. Since they spend so much time down there, and put everything they see in their mouths, it is important to keep floors as clean and uncluttered as possible.

- Teach your children not to run in your home. They could slip and fall on slick floors.
- Keep floors clear and uncluttered to prevent trips and falls.
- Wipe up spills as soon as they occur.
- Secure all area rugs with two-sided tape to prevent slips.

Kitchen

While the kitchen may be the heart of the home, it is also the most dangerous room in the home. Children can burn their

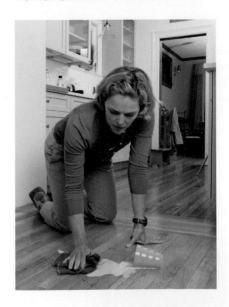

tips

Poisoning Prevention in the Kitchen.

Although under the kitchen sink seems like a convenient location for storing cleaning products, it's actually the *worst* place to store such products when you have young children. Instead, choose a cabinet high up, maybe the one over the refrigerator, to store such products. Other options include a high shelf in a hall closet near the kitchen.

Also consider switching to natural products like vinegar and baking soda for cleaning, which pose much lower poisoning risks to children.

Keep these other safety tips in mind:

- Keep all detergents, disinfectants, oven and window cleansers and drain cleaners stored away from food.
- Store all cleaning products in their original containers and make sure they're properly sealed.
- Use child safety locks on all cabinets in which poisonous products are stored—even if they're stored up high.

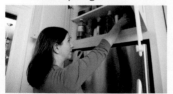

hands on hot pots and stoves, cut themselves with knives or poison themselves with cleaning supplies. Turn your kitchen from scary to safe for both you *and* your children.

Knife Safety. Many kitchen accidents are knife related, so make sure older children (those age 12 and older) know how to safely use a knife and keep knives far back on the counter where young children can't reach them. Also make sure you use child-safety locks on all kitchen cabinets and drawers that contain sharp items like knives, or dangerous chemicals, like cleaning supplies. Although it's best if your child is not in the kitchen when you're cooking, if that's impossible, you might consider maintaining one unlocked cupboard filled with safe things for your child to play with, like plastic containers or small pots, or keep him in a playpen, crib, stationary activity center or safely buckled into a high chair but always within your sight while cooking.

Stoves and Ovens. The heat from stoves and ovens, the hot food going in-and-out and on-and-off of them, all pose serious hazards for a child. To reduce the risk of injury to a child:

- Cook on back burners when possible. Children like to reach for things and may reach up to the stovetop where they can't see a burner that is turned on, burning their hands on the burner or a hot pot. They may also pull hot liquids onto themselves. Keep your child at least 3 feet away from any heat source.
- Always turn pot handles toward the back of the stove.
- Never carry hot liquids or food near your child or while holding your child.
- Use an appliance latch to keep the oven door closed, even when you're not cooking. A curious child could open the oven and climb up and into it, becoming trapped.
- Use dry potholders, not wet; wet potholders can create scalding steam.
- Do not leave surface units or burners on when unattended. Also, watch fat and grease closely so they do not become too hot and catch on fire or splatter and burn a nearby child.
- Warn children not to touch heating elements, even if they look cool.
- Do not set bowls, utensils and towels near electric units or gas burners where they could catch fire.
- Never use the oven door to stand on because the range could tip, resulting in serious burns or other injuries.
- Don't store pots or other items inside the oven.
- Do not leave hot pots or utensils where a child can touch them. If practical cool off all pots and pans before leaving them in the dishwasher or sink.
- Don't use the range to heat the room. It could overheat or lead to burns or other injuries. It can also generate carbon monoxide, a colorless, odorless gas that can cause poisoning, brain damage and

even death. (See Smoke Alarms and Carbon Monoxide Alarms, page 12.)

Refrigerators. Refrigerators always attract children; all that good food! To prevent a tragedy—

- Use a safety latch on refrigerators so children can't open the door themselves.
- Caution children not to climb, hang or stand on refrigerator or freezer shelves.
- Remove the door or door latch when disposing of a refrigerator so children can't crawl inside and become trapped.

Microwaves. Twenty years ago, few kitchens had microwaves; today, we couldn't survive without one. Even 6-year-olds often use microwaves to heat up a snack. It's important that your child know how to use the microwave safely when old enough, and equally important that you use it safely to reduce the risk of injuries to children around you. Teach your children the following tips and make sure you follow them yourself:

- Do not try to use a microwave with the door open. Some older models might start with the door open.

- Use only cooking dishes safe for the microwave, and remove all metal, including metal twist ties, from microwavable foods and dishes.
- Always use potholders to remove dishes from the microwave. The container can be hotter than it looks.
- Pierce foods like potatoes and plastic wrap coverings before microwaving to avoid explosions.
- Do not overcook food.
- Do not heat containers with small openings, like syrup bottles.
- Do not boil eggs in their shell in the microwave; they could explode.
- **NEVER** warm a bottle in a microwave; hot spots could potentially burn the baby. Instead, warm the bottle until it is lukewarm (not hot) by running it under warm faucet water or placing it in a pot or bowl of hot water.
- Stir food well after removing it from the microwave to eliminate hot spots.

Tables and Work Surfaces. The table and work surfaces in the kitchen need to be kept as clean as possible to avoid spreading germs from uncooked or undercooked food, which can result in food poisoning and other foodborne illnesses. Use a separate cutting board for uncooked meat, poultry or fish. After cutting the food, clean the board with hot, soapy water—not a sponge—or rinse and put in the dishwasher. Periodically clean with a mild bleach solution. (See also Food Safety, page 36.)

High Chairs and Infant Seats. Sometimes you have to have your baby or young child in the kitchen with you while you prepare meals. Don't let him play underfoot—you could trip while carrying a pot of hot soup. Instead, keep him secured in a high chair, booster seat, stationary play chair or infant seat, and follow this advice:

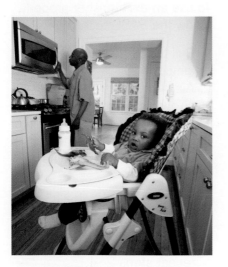

- Keep high chairs and other child seats away from the stove and other hot appliances.
- Make sure your child is buckled securely into any high chair, booster seat or other child seat. They are easy to climb and slip out of. And never leave a young child alone in the kitchen.
- Keep matches, hot liquids and foods out of children's reach, particularly when they are in a high chair and can reach up higher.
- Keep infant seats on the floor, not on a raised surface, to prevent falls. Never place an infant seat or carrier on a table or counter. The child could tip it and fall to the floor.

Fire Extinguishers. If you have the right type of fire extinguisher in the right place at the right time, you can keep a small flame from becoming a dangerous fire. But it's important that you know how to use an extinguisher in an emergency and how to maintain it. The following tips will help.

- Consider having one or more fire extinguishers in your home, including one within easy reach of the stove in the kitchen.

- Fire extinguishers rated "A-B-C" are recommended for home use. Purchase only Underwriters Laboratory (UL)- or Factory Mutual Laboratories (FML)-approved fire extinguishers and maintain them according to manufacturer's instructions.
- Get training from your local fire department or a fire extinguisher manufacturer on how to use your fire extinguisher. Not all fire extinguishers operate alike, so understanding how to use the one you have will keep you safer in the event of a fire. Remember, there is no time to read directions during an emergency and only adults should handle and use fire extinguishers.
- Fire extinguishers should be looked at regularly to ensure that they are appropriately charged. Use the gauge or test button to check that there is proper pressure. If the unit is low on pressure, damaged or corroded, replace it or have it professionally serviced.
- Before you begin to put out a fire with a fire extinguisher, be sure that—
  - Everyone has left or is leaving the home.
  - Someone has or is calling 9-1-1 or the local emergency number from a neighbor's home or cell phone.
  - The fire is small and not spreading.
  - Your back is to an exit you can use quickly.
  - There is not heavy smoke in the room.
- If the fire does not immediately die down, drop the extinguisher and get out. Most portable extinguishers empty in as little as 8 to 10 seconds.
- Back away from an extinguished fire in case it flares up.
- Once the fire extinguisher has been discharged, it should be discarded or recharged as directed by the manufacturer's recommendations.

To use an extinguisher properly, follow the PASS technique:

1. **P**ull the pin, which breaks the tamper seal.
2. **A**im the extinguisher low, pointing the nozzle (or its horn or hose) at the base of the fire.
3. **S**queeze the handle to release the extinguishing agent.
4. **S**weep from side to side at the base of the fire until it appears to be out. Watch the area. If the fire reignites, repeat steps 2–4.

Living Areas

Your children likely spend a lot of time in playrooms and family rooms. Keep these rooms safe so you can relax and your children can play safely.

Carpets.

- Cover slippery floors with carpets until your children are older.
- Use double-sided tape to secure area rugs so they don't slip.

Televisions and Video Equipment.

- Protect children from falling television sets with straps or by putting the television high enough so children can't reach it.
- Make sure the television and other similar equipment is secured properly so children can't tip it over.
- Never allow young children to operate video equipment on their own.
- Teach children never to stick items or food into openings in the television or video equipment.

Cords and Plugs.

- Only use extension cords that are UL approved.
- Don't tuck electric extension cords under rugs.

- Don't overload electrical outlets or use appliances with frayed or cracked wires.
- Use child safety plugs in all exposed electrical outlets so children can't stick their fingers or various items in the openings. They could get a shock.
- Use safety devices for surge protectors and extension cords to prevent children from gaining access to plugs.
- Extension cords should not be used as a substitute for permanent wiring.

Fireplaces, Wood Stoves and Space Heaters.

Each year, children are injured or killed, and thousands of fires ignited, as the result of improperly used fireplaces, wood stoves and space heaters. To keep you and your children safe:

- Install fireplace screens around fireplaces, and guards around radiators, hot pipes and wood-burning stoves.
- Install carbon monoxide detectors. (See Smoke Alarms and Carbon Monoxide Alarms, page 12).
- Make sure your space heater meets the latest safety standards from the Consumer Product Safety Commission, including an automatic cut-off device to turn off electric or

kerosene heaters if they tip over and guarding around the heating coils of electric heaters and the burner of kerosene heaters to prevent fires.

- Use kerosene heaters only if permitted by law in your area. Refuel kerosene heaters only outdoors and after they have cooled. Kerosene has a low flash point. If mistakenly dripped on hot surfaces, it can cause fires. Never substitute gasoline for kerosene in the heater.
- Place space heaters on a level, hard and non-flammable surface, not on rugs or carpets. Keep blankets, clothing, curtains, furniture, and anything that could get hot and catch fire at least 3 feet away from all heat sources. Plug heaters directly into the wall socket rather than using an extension cord.
- Keep doors open to the rest of your home if you are using an unvented fuel-burning space heater. This helps prevent pollutant build-up and promotes proper combustion. Follow the manufacturer's instructions to provide sufficient combustion air to prevent carbon monoxide production.
- Turn the space heater off and unplug it when you go to sleep. Never place a space heater close to any sleeping person.
- Turn the space heater off if you leave the area. Keep children and pets away from space heaters.
- Be aware that mobile homes require specially designed heating equipment. Only electric or vented fuel-fired equipment should be used.
- Have gas and kerosene space heaters inspected annually by a professional to ensure proper operation.
- Have flues and chimneys and wood stoves inspected before each heating season and cleaned if necessary to make sure they are not blocked by creosote or debris, and to check for any leaking.
- Chimneys and wood stoves build up creosote, which is the residue left behind by burning wood. Creosote is flammable and needs to be professionally removed periodically.
- Open the fireplace damper before lighting the fire and keep it open until the ashes are cool. Store ashes in a metal container with a tight-fitting lid. This will prevent the build-up of poisonous gases, especially while the family is sleeping.

- Never use gasoline, charcoal lighter or other fuel to light or relight a fire because the vapors can explode. Never keep or store flammable fuels or materials near a fire.
- Keep a fireplace screen or glass enclosure around a fireplace to prevent sparks or embers from igniting flammable materials.

Family Fire Escape Plan. It's important to have and practice an escape plan in case of a fire. Follow these tips to make sure your family is prepared and knows what to do in the event of a fire in your home.

- Draw a diagram of each floor in your home and, with your children's help, identify two ways to exit from each room.
- Place a collapsible escape ladder (meeting an Underwriter's Laboratory classification or ASTM standard) near all upper-story windows. Make sure you practice using these during fire drills from a first-story window only.
- Agree on a safe place where family members will gather away from the burning building. This safe place should be a stationary object such as the mailbox, lamppost, tree or neighbor's driveway, not something that can move or might not be there, such as a car.
- Practice your fire escape drill at least twice a year during the day and at night. If your household includes young children, or an elderly or handicapped person, make sure your escape plan includes steps to ensure their safety.
- Some children may not awaken to the sound of the smoke alarm. Know what your child will do before a fire by conducting home fire drills while children are sleeping.
- Make sure each family member understands the importance of crawling low under smoke when escaping from a burning building.
- Make sure every family member knows to get out first; then call for help.

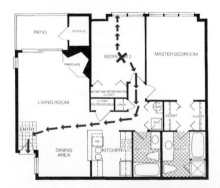

tips

Smoke Alarms and Carbon Monoxide Alarms

If you have a fire, smoke alarms can cut nearly in half your risk of dying in a fire.

- Install and maintain smoke alarms on every level of your home, outside sleeping areas and inside each bedroom. If someone in your home may not hear an alarm while sleeping, consider installing alternative alarms such as strobe lights or vibrating alarms.
- Test and dust smoke alarms once a month.
- Change the batteries in smoke alarms every year.
- Replace smoke alarms every 10 years.

Carbon monoxide, a colorless, odorless gas produced by any burning fuel, can build up in your home and bloodstream, eventually leading to death. Symptoms include aches, dizziness, headache, confusion, and other symptoms also found with flu and typical cold-weather viruses. To help prevent carbon monoxide poisoning:

- Have your furnace inspected and adjusted before every heating season.
- Have your chimney, fireplace, wood stoves and flues inspected before every heating season.
- Have chimneys and flues repaired as needed.
- Ventilate the room every time you use a kerosene space heater.
- Do not use charcoal grills indoors for cooking or heating.
- Never use gas appliances such as ranges, ovens or clothes dryers for heating your home.
- Do not leave your car's engine running in an enclosed or attached garage.

To detect carbon monoxide:

- Install a carbon monoxide alarm on every level of your home and near every sleeping area in your home.
- If the alarm sounds, get everyone out of your home and into a fresh air location. CALL 9-1-1 or the local emergency number. Remain in the fresh air location until emergency personnel say it is safe to return to your home.

Bookcases, Walkers, Playpens, Toy Boxes and Chests. Children may look little, but they can be amazingly strong—especially when it comes to their ability to pull furniture down on themselves. Keep them safe by securing bookcases and other heavy furniture to the wall and cautioning children not to climb or play on furniture. Other tips to keep your kids safe when it comes to furniture are:

- Ensure that all paint or finish on children's furniture and playpens is nontoxic.
- Do not use a baby walker that moves. More children have been injured with these items than with any other nursery product. Only put your child in seats that do not move.
- Always make sure a playpen is set up properly according to the manufacturer's directions.
- Since children may use the top rail of the playpen for teething, check the rails frequently for holes and tears.
- Don't hang toys from the sides of playpens with strings or cords because they could wrap around a child's neck.
- Never use a playpen with holes in the mesh sides. A child's head could become trapped.
- Check to see if the staples used to attach the mesh side to the floor plate are loose or missing.
- Only use playpens with hinges in the center of each of the four top rails if the top rail automatically locks when the rail is lifted into the normal use position.
- Make sure the mattress pad fits snugly and do not add a second pad or mattress. Babies could suffocate if they become trapped between mattresses or between the playpen side and a too-small mattress.
- Never leave an infant in a mesh playpen or crib with the drop-side down. Infants can roll into the space between the mattress and loose mesh and suffocate. Even when a child is not in a playpen, leave the drop-side up.
- Remove large toys, bumper pads or boxes from inside the playpen. Children could use them for climbing out.

- Ensure that slat spaces on a wooden playpen are no more than 2-⅜ inches (60 mm) in width.
- If you are using an older or used playpen, check the Consumer Product Safety Commission Web site (*www.cpsc.gov*) to see if it has been recalled.
- Make sure toy boxes have secure lids and safe-closing hinges.
- Make sure toy chests have a support that will hold the hinged lid open in any position in which it is placed or buy one with a detached lid or doors.
- Make certain that the lid of the toy chest does not have a latch.
- Look for a toy chest with ventilation holes that will not be blocked if the chest is placed against the wall or a chest that, when closed, has a gap between the lid and the sides of the chest. Many chests are ventilated by a space between the underside of the lid and sides or front of the box.
- If you already own a toy chest or trunk with a freely falling lid, remove the lid. Children have been killed when lids collapsed on their head and neck, or when they suffocated after climbing into a toy box.

- Secure all furniture so it cannot tip over.

Bedrooms

We spend more time in our bedrooms than in any other room in the home. And children, who usually sleep more than us, spend even more time in theirs. Make sure you create a safe, protected environment for them to rest in by following these tips:

Curtain Cords. Dangling curtain or blind cords can strangle a child. That's why it's so important that you keep all curtain cords and shade pulls out of children's reach. Either use tie-down devices or cut the cord in half to make two separate cords. Contact Window Covering Safety Council to get free repair kits (800-506-4634; *www.windowcoverings.org/20.html*). Also look for blinds sold with child-safe mechanisms that eliminate the risk of strangulation.

Cosmetics, Jewelry and Other Small Objects.

- Keep cosmetics, perfumes and breakable items stored out of children's reach.
- Keep small objects such as jewelry, buttons and safety pins out of children's reach.
- When caring for an infant, avoid wearing long necklaces

that could inadvertently become wrapped around the infants' neck.

Tall and Heavy Furniture.
- Cushion sharp edges of furniture with corner guards or other material.
- Keep end tables and other furniture away from windows.
- Secure furniture to the wall so it cannot tip over.

Cribs, Beds and Sleeping Areas.
The Consumer Product Safety Commission notes that more infants die every year in accidents involving cribs than with any other nursery product, while thousands are injured seriously enough to require emergency room treatment. But bedding dangers aren't limited to cribs; an infant can suffocate or become injured if you bring him into your bed. To keep a child's bed and room safe:

- Check the labeling on all cribs to make sure they meet federal safety regulations and industry voluntary standards.
- Keep beds and cribs away from radiators and other hot surfaces.
- Never place a crib near a window or dresser.
- Check an infant's crib before putting the baby down to sleep, and remove from the crib all small objects, soft bedding and other smothering risks, such as pillows, blankets, cushions and beanbags, that can wrap around or cover the face of a small child or infant. Use a firm mattress designed for a crib.
- Put infants to sleep on their back to reduce the risk of sudden infant death syndrome (SIDS).
- Never place your infant to sleep on an adult bed, waterbed or bunk bed. Infants up to 18 months can suffocate in their sleep when their bodies or faces become wedged between the mattress and bed frame or the mattress and wall.
- Never tie pacifiers and teethers around your child's neck, and remove bibs and necklaces whenever you put your baby in a crib or playpen.
- Always lock the side rail in its raised position whenever you place your child in the crib. As

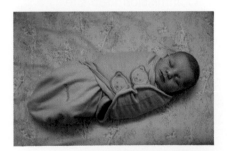

soon as your child can stand up, adjust the mattress to its lowest position and remove the bumper pads. Also, remove any large toys—an active toddler will use anything for climbing out of the crib.

- Check all crib hardware; tighten all nuts, bolts and screws frequently. After a crib is moved, be sure all mattress support hangers are secure and check hooks regularly to be sure none are broken or bent.
- Install crib gyms securely at both ends so they cannot be pulled down into the crib; remove them from the crib when your baby is 5 months old or begins to push up on hands and knees.
- Do not use crib toys with catch points that can hook clothing.
- Do not use older-model cribs or used cribs for your infant. If you have one, check the Consumer Product Safety Commission Web site (*www.cpsc.gov*) to see if it has been recalled.
- Use a guardrail on beds until a child is at least 35 inches tall.
- Do not allow a child younger than age 6 to sleep in the top bed of bunk beds.

Windows, Screens and Window Guards. Every year, thousands of young children are killed or injured in falls from windows. Take the following steps to help prevent these tragedies:

- Keep windows locked when they are closed.
- Never let children open windows by themselves, and know that screens don't prevent falls.
- Prevent windows from opening more than 4 inches by using window guards (with the exception of a fire escape window).
- Keep windows and doors to the outside locked, and install childproof latches and window guards on all windows and balcony doors.

Toys. Most babies or toddlers like to put anything they can get their hands on into their mouths, so follow these tips to keep them safe when they're playing with their toys:

- Make sure all toys are in good repair.
- Ensure all toys are appropriate for your child's age.
- Do not allow young children to play with ropes, cords or toys with long pull strings.

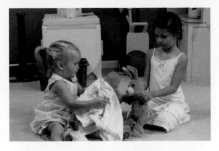

- Make sure toys are too large to be swallowed and that toys do not have small parts that can be pulled off. For infants and toddlers, in general, no toy should be smaller than 1¾ inches in diameter. Most toys are labeled and will clearly say if the toy is safe for the age group.
- Check all rattles, squeeze toys and teethers for small ends that could extend into the back of the baby's mouth, take all these toys out of the baby's crib while he is sleeping and avoid rattles and squeeze toys with ball-shaped ends.

Bathrooms

Two words come to mind when thinking of the hazards of bathrooms: water and electricity. The two don't mix with each other, and they don't mix with kids. They're not the only hazards in the bathroom and laundry room, however. Read on to discover how to reduce the risk of injury to children in these rooms.

- Keep hair dryers and other appliances unplugged and stored away from the sink, tub or toilet.
- Place safety covers on all unused electrical outlets.
- Secure loose electrical cords and do not use multi-cord plugs.
- Store all medicines in their original, child-resistant containers in a locked medicine cabinet.
- Keep razors, razor blades and other sharp objects in a locked medicine cabinet.
- Equip all cabinets with safety latches and keep them closed.
- Dispose of outdated products as recommended.
- Keep bathroom doors closed if you have small children at home.
- Install nonslip surfacing on the bottom of the tub or shower.
- Make sure an adult watches young children any time they are in the bathroom, even if they're not taking a bath. Never be more than an arm's length away from a young child taking a bath.
- Before putting your child in a tub of water, check the bath water temperature with your elbow to be sure it is not too hot.

- Be aware of any sharp edges on the faucet and keep the child's head away from it. Put a cover over the faucet.
- Keep shampoos and cosmetics stored out of children's reach.
- Keep the toilet seat and lid down when the toilet is not in use and install safety locks on toilets.

Laundry Areas. Whether your home has a laundry room big enough to wash an NFL team's clothes, or a washer/dryer hidden in a closet, follow these tips to keep the area safe when children are out and about:

- Keep laundry detergents and dryer sheets in a locked cabinet. If that isn't possible, keep them on a high shelf children can't reach. *Don't* keep them on top of the washer or dryer.
- Empty cleaning buckets immediately after use.
- Keep boxes and stools away from laundry sinks. Children could use them to climb up and fall in.
- Don't soak anything in laundry tubs if small children are home.
- Save your ironing for the evenings when children are asleep or the days when they're not home. It's too easy for young children to become entangled in the iron cord and get burned.
- Always cool hot irons in a location that children can't access.
- Make sure your ironing board is securely locked in place and won't fall while you iron.
- Put away the ironing board and iron as soon as you finish ironing.

Garages and Basements

Garages and basements draw children like bees to honey. But since most of us tend to store chemicals, paints, sharp tools and other potentially dangerous items there, they can be accidents waiting to happen. Follow these tips to childproof your basement and garage.

Automotive Tools, Fuels and Hazardous Substances.

- Unplug all power tools and, if possible, cover sharp edges or put away in a locked cabinet that children can't access.
- Don't store chemicals in food or drink containers. Keep all hazardous materials in their original containers in a locked cabinet out of reach of children.
- Keep children away when using any chemicals that could cause burns or toxic fumes.

- Keep chemicals in a locked cabinet out of the reach of children.
- Only store gasoline in a ventilated area, in a container designed especially for gasoline. And keep children away from the area.
- If you have an automatic garage door opener, make sure it is equipped with safety features so it automatically stops if a child or someone else is beneath it. Test it periodically according to the manufacturer's directions to make sure it works.
- Keep the remote opener for the automatic garage door away from children and don't let them play with it.

Shelving and Storage.
- Put shelving up high enough so children can't reach it.
- Attach shelving securely to the wall, ideally to the wall studs.
- Lock all cabinets that contain hazardous chemicals or tools.

Water Heaters and Furnaces.
- Keep children away from water heaters and furnaces. They could get burned.
- Set the maximum water heater temperature at 120° F to avoid potential scalds in children from faucet water.

- If you have a gas water heater, consider having an automatic gas shutoff valve installed that shuts down the gas flow in an emergency.
- Test the safety relief valve on your water heater annually. This valve prevents too much pressure building up in the heater, and keeps the water from exceeding 120° F.
- Keep the area around your furnace clean and free of combustible and flammable material.
- Do not close off more than 20 percent of the registers in your home. This can cause high resistance and unnecessary heat to build up in the furnace.
- Have your furnace and water heater serviced annually to ensure both are in good working condition.

Outside in the Yard and Garden
Children need fresh air and exercise, and what could be better than your yard and garden? Take a careful look around first, however, to assess any potential risks so you can keep your children safe and playing happily.

Decks.
- Make sure the slats on your deck are too small for a child

to get through; if not, install barriers.

- Check your deck annually for splintering or popped nails.
- Make sure children always wear shoes when playing on a deck.
- Keep walkways, stairs and railings in good repair and install safety gates at the top and bottom of all outside stairs.
- Keep walkways and stairs free of toys, tools and other objects.

Lawn and Garden Equipment.

- Never hold a child on your lap or allow anyone to ride as a passenger on a riding mower or in a lawn cart. Don't allow a child on or near a lawn mower when it is in use.
- Never permit a child to walk alongside, in front of or behind a moving mower.
- Don't allow a child to play on or around a lawn mower, even when it's not in use—lawn mowers aren't toys.
- Before mowing the grass, remove stones, tree branches, nails and wires from areas being mowed—these objects can be picked up by the mower and expelled, causing serious injury to a nearby child.

Pool Areas and Hot Tubs.

Children younger than age 5 and young adults from ages 15 to 24 have the highest rates of drowning. Most young children who drown do so in home pools. Thus, it is very important that you take steps to keep children out of pool areas and hot tubs if there is no adult present and safe when they're splashing around.

- If you have a pool, learn to swim—and be sure everyone in the household knows how to swim. Enroll your children in an American Red Cross Learn-to-Swim class (*www.redcross.org*). Parents should take a Red Cross water safety course.
- Watch children continuously around any water no matter how well your child can swim or how shallow the water, and never use flotation devices and inflatable toys as a substitute for adult supervision.

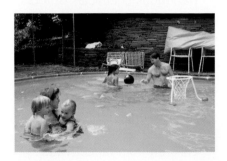

- Stay within an arm's reach of an inexperienced swimmer while he or she is in the water.
- Empty kiddie pools immediately after use. This prevents a toddler or young child from falling in and, possibly, drowning.
- Never leave unattended a child who may gain access to any water.
- Teach your child never to go near the water without you; the pool area is off limits without adult supervision.
- Enclose the pool completely with a fence that has vertical bars and a self-closing, self-latching gate. Openings in the fence should be no more than 4 inches wide and your home should not be part of the barrier. However, if your home *is* part of the barrier, install an additional fence and keep the doors and windows leading from your home to the pool locked and protected with an alarm that sounds when the door is unexpectedly opened.
- Prevent access to garden water features, such as ponds and waterfalls.
- Never leave furniture or toys where a child could use them to climb over the fence to gain access to the pool. Also, keep toys that might attract young children away from the pool when not in use.
- Always remove pool covers completely prior to pool use and ensure they are completely secured when in place.
- Keep the pool water clean and clear.
- Keep a telephone near the pool or bring a fully charged cordless or mobile phone poolside and post 9-1-1 or the local emergency number as well as your address and the nearest cross streets so that anyone can read them to an emergency dispatcher.
- Always keep basic lifesaving equipment, such as a reaching pole, rope and flotation devices, by the pool and know how to use them.
- Post cardiopulmonary resuscitation (CPR) and first aid instructions in the pool area and keep a well-stocked first aid kit available.
- If a child is missing, check the pool first. Scan the entire pool, bottom and surface, as well as the surrounding pool area.
- Do not allow children younger than 5 years of age into a spa or hot tub.
- Never allow unsupervised children to use a spa or hot tub.

tips

Sun Safety

Luckily, you can have fun in the sun while protecting yourself and your children from harmful UV rays.

Make sure to wear sunscreen, even on a cloudy day. You can still get burned when it's cloudy. The sun's rays are strongest between 10 a.m. and 4 p.m. During these hours, avoid exposure to the sun or seek shade, if possible.

Apply sunscreen 20 minutes before you and your children go outside. Reapply every 2 hours and after swimming or sweating.

Make sure the sunscreen has a sun protection factor (SPF) of at least 15 and preferably 30 or higher.

For infants, use only sunscreen that is recommended for use on infants. When putting sunscreen on infants younger than 6 months old, apply a small amount on the face and the back of the hands, although adequate clothing and shade are preferable.

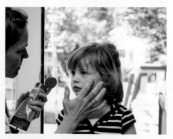

- Make sure the water temperature in a hot tub or spa does not exceed 104° F.
- If children are old enough to use a spa, limit their time spent in one to 15 minutes or less.
- After using a spa, make your children wait at least 5 minutes before swimming. A sudden change in temperature can cause problems.
- Test and treat your spa or hot tub regularly to prevent bacteria and parasite growth.
- Make sure your pool or spa has a safety vacuum release and anti-entrapment drain cover to prevent suction entrapment, and replace the drain immediately if it does not.
- Know the location of the emergency cut-off switch for your spa.
- Securely cover a hot tub or spa when not in use.
- Store pool chemicals in childproof containers and out of children's reach.

Swing Sets, Jungle Gyms and Sandboxes. It's so easy today to create an almost instant-playground in your own back yard. But it's important to purchase playground equipment that meets the latest safety standards and that the equipment is installed properly and in good condition. Always supervise children at all times when they're playing on the equipment. Also check the following:

- Repair sharp points or edges on equipment. Replace missing hardware and close "S" hooks that can cause injuries.
- Never attach ropes, jump ropes, clotheslines, pet leashes or cords of any kind to play equipment due to the strangulation hazard.
- Look for openings or railings that could trap a child's hands, head or feet. Any space larger than the width of a soda can is unsafe.
- Dress your child for play. That means no clothes with drawstrings and hoods that could catch on equipment.
- Check for sand, wood chips or rubber matting under play equipment to cushion children's falls.
- Check that the sand in sandboxes is clean and free of glass and debris.
- If you see any sharp objects on the equipment, such as rusty nails or splinters, clear them off and throw them away.

- Make sure the equipment is the right size for your child. For instance, only school-age children should use jungle gyms higher than 30 inches off the ground, and the equipment should have guardrails or barriers.
- Make sure rungs, stairs and steps are evenly spaced, with spaces between them less than 3-½ inches wide or more than 9 inches wide so a child's head doesn't get caught.
- Round rungs on jungle gyms should be about 1 to 1-½ inches around.
- Swings should be clear of any other equipment with enough room in front and behind it for swinging, and seats should be made of soft materials, such as rubber, plastic or canvas, not wood.
- Make sure swings are not too close together. They should be at least 2 feet apart with no more than two seat swings in the same part of the set.

Outdoor Pests and Animals and Poisonous Plants. We might go outside, but animals and insects call the outside their home. So make sure your children are prepared to share the outdoors with those winged and furry residents without any ill effects.

- Spray insect repellent containing diethyltoluamide (DEET) on children when they go into grassy or wooded areas or if you know the area is infested with insects or ticks. Only use products that contain less than 10 percent DEET and consult your pediatrician before using these products on a younger child.
- Dress children in light-colored long pants tucked into socks and a long-sleeved shirt to help protect them against mosquitoes and ticks and to make ticks easier to spot.
- Check for ticks when your child has been in grassy or wooded areas.
- Make sure there is no standing water in your yard, such as water in buckets and stagnant ponds or birdbaths. Mosquitoes breed in standing water.
- Keep food and the trashcan covered at picnics. Sweet foods and drinks attract bees and wasps.
- Make sure your children wear shoes at all times outdoors, even if they're playing in grass.
- Teach children to stay away from beehives and wasp nests and not to swat bees or wasps with their hands.

Children should stand still and the insects should go away.
- Check the area for poisonous plants (your local poison control center can provide information on poisonous plants specific to your area). Also check for plants with thorns, stickers and roots that stick up and trees with low branches that could cause scratches.

Safety Outside the Home

Once you get out of your own backyard, you lose a certain amount of control over your environment. However, there are still things you can do to make sure your child remains safe and secure, whether at the park or on a shopping trip with you.

Playgrounds

According to the Consumer Product Safety Commission, about 200,000 children each year are treated in hospital emergency rooms for injuries related to playground equipment. When you arrive at a playground, do a quick check for rough spots, holes and any objects that could trip children. Also follow these safety rules when using the play equipment in your backyard (see also

Swing Sets, Jungle Gyms and Sandboxes, page 22). Remember to do the following:

- Always supervise children on play equipment to make sure they are safe.
- Check whether protective surfacing, including shredded/recycled rubber, wood chips, wood mulch, sand or pea gravel, is under and around playground equipment to cushion children from falls. It should be at least 9 inches deep.
- Check that protective surfacing extends at least 6 feet in all directions from play equipment. The protective surfacing should extend in front and back of swings, twice the height of the suspending bar.
- Check for trash; broken glass or cement; needles; animal droppings; sewage; and shiny objects, like open aluminum cans, which may be sharp and can cause wounds.

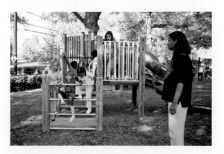

- Check that restrooms are clean and safe for children, but do not leave the children alone when you inspect a restroom. Make sure to check the restroom for people. If anyone looks suspicious, leave the restroom and don't allow children to go into restrooms by themselves.
- Watch out for loose animals.
- Watch out for storm drains and keep children away from them, especially after a rainstorm.
- Check for any water in the area, such as a fountain, pond or lake. Do not allow children to play near the water unless you are within arm's reach of them.
- Check for any moving parts that might pinch or trap a child or child's body part.
- Make sure wooden equipment is free of nails and splinters.
- Check the surface of slides to make sure they are not too hot. Also make sure they have a platform at the top with guardrails.
- Check the base of the slide for rocks, sticks, animal droppings or other debris that could harm a child.
- Always watch your children as they are playing, and be particularly wary of any strangers in the area who try to approach your child.

Shopping Malls and Grocery Stores

According to the Consumer Product Safety Commission, more than 20,000 children a year are treated for injuries related to shopping carts. Keep your child safe with these tips:

- If you can, avoid shopping carts. They tip over easily and are just not designed for carrying small children. If you have no other option, make sure your child is restrained.
- Never allow your child to stand up in the cart or ride on the outside.
- Never leave a child alone in the cart.
- Keep your child close by at all times and do not let him wander off.
- If you're going to a very crowded store, such as a shopping mall during the holidays, pin a note to your child with his name and your name and cell phone number in case you are separated.

Public Pools

Follow these tips so that you can provide an extra layer of protection for your children while at a public pool:

- Teach your child how to swim before you head for the neighborhood pool. The Red

Cross has swimming courses for children of any age and swimming ability. To enroll in a swimming course, contact your local Red Cross chapter.
- Teach your children to enter the water feet first. They should enter head-first only when the area is clearly marked for diving and has no obstructions.
- Teach your children to walk, not run, at the pool. Running on slippery concrete is a sure way to trip and fall.
- Have your children wear footwear at the pool. The concrete can get very hot during the day and burn young feet.
- Watch your children continuously around any water no matter how well your children can swim or how shallow the water is.
- Stay within an arm's reach of an inexperienced swimmer while he or she is in the water.
- Never use flotation devices and inflatable toys as a substitute for adult supervision.

Daycares

Choosing a daycare provider is one of the most important decisions you will make for your children. Make sure the provider is licensed, trained and well versed in children's health and safety issues and that the environment meets your expectations. Visit the National Resource Center for Health and Safety in Child Care and Early Education's Web site (*http://nrc.uchsc.edu/CFOC*) for more information on national health and safety performance standards and guidelines for out-of-home child care programs in all 50 states and U.S. territories.

Vehicle Safety

People are often scared of taking an airplane trip, but the truth is that the most dangerous trip you take is in your car, and the primary cause of injuries and death in young children is related to vehicles. You can keep your child safe in your car and out of it with the following advice:

- Make sure all children wear safety belts, including a shoulder restraint, even if you're just going around the corner for milk.
- Always place infants in a rear-facing safety seat in the backseat until they are at least 1 year old and 20 pounds. Children 1 year of age and at least 20 pounds may ride in a forward-facing seat in the backseat;

however, it is best for them to ride rear-facing until they reach the weight and height limits of the seat. Ask your local fire department, emergency medical service personnel or hospital to show you how to install the child safety seat properly. They should have a National Highway Transportation Safety Administration-trained car safety seat technician advise you.

- Keep toddlers and preschoolers in a forward-facing seat with a harness until they have reached about 40 pounds and are about 4 years old.

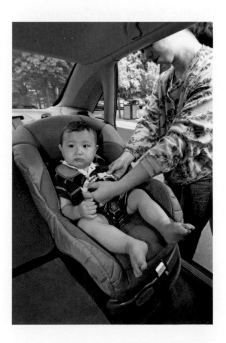

- When they have outgrown their forward-facing seats, have children ride in a booster seat until an adult seat belt fits them properly, typically when a child reaches 4'9" in height and is 8–12 years old.
- Always have children younger than age 13 sit in the rear, away from air bags, wearing a seat belt.
- Don't leave objects like toys and other items loose in your car. If an accident occurs, they could become high-speed missiles.
- Do not drink and drive! Doing so puts you and your children—as well as other people—at serious risk.

Traffic Safety and Crossing the Street. Teach safety rules to your children for crossing the street, including:

- Holding hands with an adult when crossing the street.
- Looking both ways before crossing.
- Crossing only at the crosswalk.
- Only crossing the street with a grown-up or other responsible adult.

Bicycling. Bicycling is fun and it's a great aerobic activity to support a healthy lifestyle. The best way to teach your children safe cycling skills is to model this behavior yourself. So make sure everyone in your family—including adults—follows these important bicycle safety rules:

- When cycling, always wear an approved helmet. The head or neck is the most seriously injured part of the body in most fatally injured cyclists.
- Be sure the helmet meets standards set by the Consumer Product Safety Commission, the Snell Memorial Foundation, the American Society for Testing and Materials or the American National Standards Institute. Look for a label or a sticker on the box or inside the helmet for this certification.

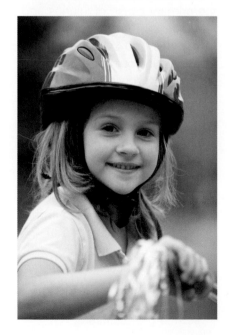

- Make sure the helmet is the correct size, is positioned correctly (level) on the head and that chin straps are properly adjusted and fastened. Check the helmet every 6 months to make sure it still fits properly.
- Children should wear a helmet even if they are still riding along the sidewalk on training wheels. Some states have helmet laws that apply to young children.
- Be sure children wear closed shoes when riding a bicycle.
- Keep your children's bicycles in good condition. Check brakes and tire pressure before each ride.
- Keep off busy roads without shoulders.
- Only older children should be able to cycle at night, and then only if they wear reflective clothing and if their bikes have a headlight, taillight and reflectors.
- Teach older children the rules of the road before allowing them to ride in the street.

Scooters, Skateboards, Inline Skates, ATVs and Other Riding Toys.
Kids love outside toys, particularly toys that help them move faster than their own two legs. But with speed comes the potential for injury. Keep your kids safe—no matter what their preferred mode of transportation—with these suggestions:

- Show your children how to use a helmet properly. It should be tightly buckled, with the front stopping just over the eyebrows. Check their helmets every 6 months to ensure they still fit.
- The best helmets for riding toys are those meeting standards set by the Consumer Product Safety Commission, the Snell Memorial Foundation, the American Society for Testing and Materials (ATSM) or the American National Standards Institute (ANSI). Look for proof on the label.
- Make sure children wear protective gear, including a helmet, knee and elbow pads and wrist guards, before hopping on a skateboard or scooter or buckling on their in-line skates. Children who do "tricks" with the skateboard should also wear gloves.
- Warn your children never to hold onto the back of a moving vehicle while riding a skateboard or scooter, or while skating.

- Make sure children use riding toys only on smooth, flat surfaces so they can maintain control.
- Don't let children use any riding toy after dark.
- Train children to use their riding toys away from traffic. For instance, parks are best for in-line skating, scooters and skateboards, while protected bike paths or sidewalks are best for the two-wheeled riding toys.
- Limit the use of four-wheeled, all-terrain vehicles (ATVs) to those who have a driver's license. Three-wheeled ATVs should never be ridden. They are unsafe and should never be used by riders of any age.
- ATVs should only be used off road—never on streets designed for vehicles.
- Never let your child drive an ATV after dark, and make sure the vehicle is festooned with flags, reflectors and lights to make it more visible.
- If your children use ATVs, make sure they have:
  - Seat belts and a roll bar. The roll bar is important because if the vehicle rolls over, the driver is not crushed by its weight.
  - Headlights that automatically turn on when the engine starts to improve visibility.
  - Speed governors, which are devices that limit maximum speed.
- Don't let your children carry anyone in their ATV and don't let your children ride in someone else's ATV.
- ATV riders should wear motorcycle (not bicycle) helmets with safety visors, eye protection and protective reflective clothing.

Strangers and Separation

You want to keep your child safe, but you don't want him to lose his inborn sense of trust. So how do you warn him about strangers? And if you tell him to never talk to strangers, then what happens if you become separated in a crowd? Try these suggestions:

- Decide what information you want to share with your child before you sit down to talk about strangers. Be sure you can answer the following questions: Who is a stranger? Are all strangers dangerous? Are there any strangers that I can talk with? What should I do when I see a stranger?
- Teach your children about which strangers he can talk to, "safe strangers" such as police and firefighters in

uniform, teachers and counselors from their school, or store managers or other authority figures if he becomes separated from you or lost.

- Explain to your child that a stranger is someone you don't know, even if they *say* they know you, your family or other people who know you. Even if someone knows your name, if you don't know them, or your parent didn't tell you about them, that person is a stranger and you should not speak or go with them.
- Teach your child that if an adult is bothering him or following him, he should find another adult immediately.
- Teach your child never to open the door to strangers and always to check through a peephole or window before opening the door. This applies to delivery people or service representatives, unless you have told them otherwise. If you do want an older child to allow a service representative in your home, make sure the child asks for identification first and reads it carefully.
- Never allow strangers to give children gifts. Have the stranger give the gift to you and then you can give the gift to your child. Establish this as a rule.

- Tell your child just as much as he needs to hear based on his age. For instance, 2 year olds view the world quite differently than do 5 year olds. Base the information you provide on your child's personality and maturity level, but don't overdo it and needlessly frighten your child.
- Bring up the subject of strangers regularly within conversation. For instance, if you are watching television with your child and you see a situation in which a stranger approaches a child, use that as a learning experience.
- Listen to your child's concerns about strangers. Ask him if he has any questions, and answer them honestly.
- Role play with your child. For instance, pretend you're the stranger; how will your child react when approached? Afterwards, sit down and discuss what went right and what didn't, and what changes can be made next time.
- Identify "safe places" your child should go to when you're out together if you get separated, such as the customer service counter, security desk or checkout counter in a store. If you are

in an outside location, identify a meeting place when you arrive, such as a fountain or statue, in case you get separated.

- Make sure your child knows your cell phone number. If your child is young, you may want to put a copy of it in his pocket.

Keeping Your Child Healthy

Keeping your child healthy means more than avoiding accidents. It also means avoiding germs that can lead to illnesses. Many of the steps required to avoid illnesses are simple—like hand washing.

Proper Hand Washing

- You and your children should wash your hands with soap and warm water for at least 15 seconds after using the toilet, when they get home from school, before eating, after touching an animal, after blowing their nose, sneezing or coughing, and before going to bed.
- Use these instructions to teach your children proper hand-washing technique:
  - Turn on warm water.
  - Wet your hands with water and put soap on your hands.

- Rub your hands together for at least 15 seconds (about the time it takes to sing "Happy Birthday" once).
- Scrub your nails by rubbing them against the palms of your hands.
- Rinse your hands with water.
- In a public restroom, dry your hands with a paper towel and turn off the faucet using the paper towel. Throw the paper towel away.
- Alcohol-based hand sanitizers can be a good alternative to washing your hands if there is no soap and water available and your hands don't have visible dirt or blood on them.
- To use an alcohol-based hand sanitizer:
  - Apply the hand sanitizer to the palm of one hand, using the amount recommended by the manufacturer.
  - Rub hands together making sure to cover all surfaces of the hands and fingers until they are dry.
- Remember always to supervise young children when using an alcohol-based hand sanitizer and keep it out of the reach of children.

Germs

Germs often come from direct contact with other people's body fluids, such as blood and saliva. Other ways germs are transmitted include:

- Breathing in droplets from someone else's cough or sneeze.
- Contact with an object or surface that has been in contact with a germ, such as a telephone.
- An insect, animal or human bite.

To reduce the spread of germs, teach children to cough or sneeze into a tissue. If a tissue is not available, show children how to use the crook of their elbow or their upper arm, keeping germs off their hands where they spread easier. Follow this advice yourself!

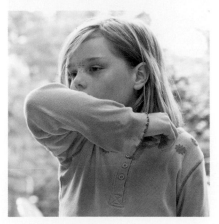

The best way to avoid the germs of others is with hand washing. If you might come into contact with blood or other body fluids, such as urine or vomit, consider using disposable gloves.

Colds

The best way to avoid a cold is by avoiding germs. Follow these suggestions:

- Keep toys clean. Every couple of days—more often if anyone in your home is sick—wipe off toys with a non-bacterial wipe, or wash in a sink of warm, soapy water.
- Keep trash out of the reach of children.
- Make sure your family eats healthy, gets plenty of rest and exercises regularly. These three things are the best way to help your body fight off infection.

Fevers

Young children can go from a perfectly normal temperature to a high fever in what seems like minutes. Don't panic! Fever is a sign that the body is working to get rid of the germs causing the illness. Fever occurs when a child's or an infant's body temperature rises above normal. A fever is defined as a temperature of 100.4° F or greater.

However, infants younger than 3 months with any fever (temperature over 100.4° F) and children under 2 years old with a high fever (103° F) typically require immediate evaluation by a physician.

If you think your child has a fever, use the right type of thermometer. A rectal temperature is recommended for children under age 5, and an oral temperature (in the mouth) for children age 5 and older. You can also use a tympanic thermometer to take the temperature in the ear or you can take it under the arm, called the axillary method.

If your child has a fever, you can use acetaminophen or ibuprofen in children older than 6 months (as advised by your pediatrician) to bring it down. For more on what to do if your child has a fever, see Fever, page 86.

IMPORTANT: Never give aspirin to a child with a fever. It could cause a rare but potentially fatal illness called Reye's syndrome.

Poisoning

A poison is any substance that can cause injury, illness or death when it gets into the body. Poisons can enter the body by ingestion (drinking or eating the poison), inhalation (breathing the poison in), absorption (the poison enters through the skin) or injection (the poison is injected into the body).

If a child is sick and you don't know why, look for items like open or spilled containers, medicines or plants nearby. This can give you clues that a poisoning has happened.

If you suspect that a child is showing signals of poisoning, CALL the National Poison Control Center (PCC) hotline at (800) 222-1222. If the child is unconscious, there is a change in the level of consciousness or if another life-threatening

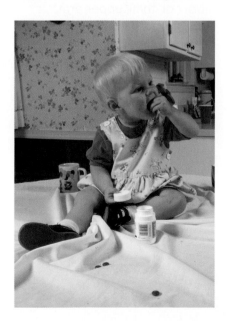

condition is present, CALL
9-1-1 or the local emergency
number right away. (See
Poisoning, page 98.)

Poisoning Prevention. Take the
following steps to keep your
children safe from poisoning:

- Always supervise children
  closely, especially in areas
  where poisons are commonly
  stored, such as kitchens,
  bathrooms, laundry rooms
  and garages.
- Keep all medications and
  household products locked
  away, well out of reach of
  children.
- Install special clamps to keep
  children from opening
  cabinets.
- Consider all household or
  drugstore products to be
  potentially harmful.
- Use child-resistant safety
  caps on medicine containers
  and other potentially
  dangerous products.
- Never call medicine "candy"
  to get a child to take it, even
  if it has a pleasant candy
  flavor.
- Keep products in their
  original containers with the
  labels in place.
- Use poison symbols to
  identify dangerous
  substances and teach children
  what the symbols mean.

- If your home was built before
  1977, you may have lead
  paint. As paint ages, it chips,
  peels and comes off as lead
  dust. Young children may
  taste or eat the dust or paint
  chips. Take the following
  steps to keep your child safe
  from lead poisoning:
  - Clean up areas that may
    have lead paint, chips or
    dust with water and
    detergent. Also keep
    surfaces like floors,
    window areas and porches
    clean to reduce your child's
    risk of exposure to lead
    dust. Rinse the sponges
    and mop heads after
    cleaning dirty or dusty
    areas.
  - Wash children's hands
    often, including before they
    eat and before going to
    sleep.
  - Keep play areas clean.
    Wash bottles, pacifiers,
    toys and stuffed animals
    regularly.
  - Keep children from
    chewing window sills or
    other painted surfaces.
  - Make sure children eat
    healthy meals. Children
    who have good nutrition
    and proper diets absorb
    less lead.
  - Have your home tested for
    lead paint and, if any is

tips

Common House Plants

Every year, people come into contact with poisonous plants such as poison ivy, poison oak and poison sumac. If your child comes into contact with these plants:

- Remove exposed clothing and wash the exposed area thoroughly with soap and water as soon as possible after contact.
- Wash clothing exposed to plant oils since the oils can linger on fabric.
- Wash your hands thoroughly after handling exposed clothing and touching exposed pets.
- Put a paste of baking soda and water on the area several times a day if a rash or weeping sore has already begun to develop. Calamine lotion and anti-histamines may also help dry up the sores and relieve itching.
- See a health-care provider if the condition gets worse. The provider may decide to give anti-inflammatory drugs such as corticosteroids or other medications to relieve discomfort.

found, a professional can recommend what you should do about it.
- Contact the National Lead Information Center for information about lead hazards and their prevention—(800)-424-5323.

Food Safety

Illness can also come from improperly prepared food or food left out too long, allowing the growth of bacteria and other pathogens. Don't let your cooking make your family sick! Instead, follow these tips:

- Wash your hands before and after handling food.
- Wash raw fruits and vegetables carefully before eating them or feeding them to children.
- Put unfinished food away in the refrigerator as soon as a meal is over. Discard any food that has been on a child or parent's plate even if it untouched. Bacteria from the fork could have been transferred to the uneaten food.

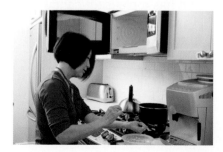

- Always test the temperature of food and drinks before giving them to children.
- Do not put hot foods like soup in the refrigerator. Allow them to cool to room temperature, or cool them in an ice bath, before refrigerating or freezing.
- Do not thaw meats at room temperature, only in the refrigerator or under cold water. If using the cold-water method, place food in a leak-proof plastic bag. Submerge in cold tap water and change the water every 30 minutes. Cook immediately after thawing. If thawed in the refrigerator, it may be refrozen before or after cooking.
- Use smooth cutting boards made of hard maple or a nonporous material such as plastic. Make sure the board is free of cracks and crevices and avoid boards made of soft, porous materials.
- Wash cutting boards with hot water, soap and a scrub brush to remove food particles. Then sanitize the boards by putting them through the automatic dishwasher or rinsing them in a solution of 1 teaspoon of chlorine bleach in 1 quart of water.
- Always wash and sanitize cutting boards after using them for raw foods and before using them for ready-to-eat foods. Consider using one cutting board only for foods that will be cooked, such as raw fish, and another only for ready-to-eat foods, such as bread, fresh fruit and cooked fish. Disposable cutting boards are a newer option and can be found in grocery and discount chain stores. After cutting raw meats, wash utensils and countertops with hot, soapy water. Utensils and countertops also can be sanitized by using a solution of 1 tablespoon of unscented, liquid chlorine bleach in 1 gallon of water.
- When shopping, buy refrigerated or cold items at the end of the trip after buying all your non-perishables.
- Make sure the meat and poultry you buy is in packaging that is not torn or leaking.
- Do not buy food past the "sell-by", "use by" or other expiration dates.
- Always refrigerate perishable food within 2 hours (1 hour when the temperature is above 90° F).
- Check the temperature of your refrigerator and freezer with an appliance thermometer. The refrigerator should be at 40° F or below and the freezer at 0° F or below.

- Cook or freeze fresh poultry, fish, ground meats and variety meats within 2 days; other beef, veal, lamb or pork, within 3 to 5 days.
- Perishable food such as meat and poultry should be wrapped securely to maintain quality and to prevent meat juices from getting onto other food.
- To maintain quality when freezing meat and poultry in its original package, wrap the package again with freezer-safe foil or plastic wrap.
- Don't cross-contaminate. Keep raw meat, poultry, fish and their juices away from other food.
- Marinate meat and poultry in a covered dish in the refrigerator.
- Cook meat and poultry immediately after microwave thawing.
- Cook meats to the proper temperature.
- When serving food on a buffet, make sure hot food is held at 140° F or warmer and cold food at 40° F or colder. Use chafing dishes, slow cookers and warming trays to keep food hot. Keep food cold by nesting dishes in bowls of ice or use small serving trays and replace them often.
- Perishable food should not be left out for more than 2 hours at room temperature (1 hour when the temperature is above 90° F).
- Discard any cooked food left out at room temperature for more than 2 hours (1 hour if the temperature is above 90° F).
- Place food into shallow containers and immediately put in the refrigerator or freezer.
- Use cooked leftovers within 4 days.

Secondhand Smoke

You know that smoking is bad for your health. But did you know that secondhand smoke could also harm your child's health? It's composed of hundreds of dangerous chemicals and has been linked to cancer, respiratory infections, bronchitis and pneumonia. Secondhand smoke also increases the risk of ear infections and asthma in young children. In fact, exposure to smoke from 10 cigarettes per day may put children at risk of developing asthma. Smoking also increases the risk of fires and burns to your children.

So if you or anyone else in your household smokes, talk to your health-care professional about steps you can take to quit. And until you do, take the smoke outside, away from the kids.

Home Safety Checklist

To Prevent Wounds. Make sure that:

- [ ] Knives, hand tools, power tools, razor blades, scissors and other objects that can cause injury are stored in locked cabinets or locked storage areas.
- [ ] Guns are stored unloaded in a locked place out of reach of children, with the ammunition stored in a separate locked place.

To Prevent Falls. Make sure that:

- [ ] Safety gates are installed at all open stairways in homes with small children and infants.
- [ ] Windows and balcony doors have childproof latches or window guards.
- [ ] Balconies have protective barriers to prevent children from slipping through the bars.
- [ ] Your home is free of clutter on the floors, especially on or near stairways.

To Prevent Poisoning. Make sure that:

- [ ] Potential poisons, like detergents, polishes, pesticides, car-care fluids, lighter fluids and lamp oils are stored in locked cabinets and are out of reach of children.

- [ ] Houseplants are kept out of reach.
- [ ] Medicine is kept in a locked storage place that children can't reach.
- [ ] Child-resistant packaging is closed or reclosed securely.

To Prevent Burns. Make sure that:

- [ ] Safety covers are placed on all unused electrical outlets.
- [ ] Loose electrical cords are secured and out of the way.
- [ ] Multi-cord plugs, also known as "octopus plugs," are not used.
- [ ] At least one approved smoke alarm is installed and operating on each level of the home.
- [ ] Space heaters are placed out of the reach of children and away from curtains.
- [ ] Flammable liquids are securely stored in their original containers and away from heat.
- [ ] Matches and lighters are stored out of the reach of children.
- [ ] Garbage and recycling materials are stored in covered containers.

To Prevent Drowning. Make sure that:

☐ Swimming pools and hot tubs are completely enclosed with a barrier, such as a locked fence or gate, and covered.
☐ Wading pools and bathtubs are emptied when not in use.
☐ Toilet seats and lids are kept down when not in use.
☐ Bathroom doors are kept closed at all times.
☐ Buckets or other containers with standing water are securely covered or emptied of water.
☐ Children are supervised at all times around water.

To Prevent Choking and Other Breathing Emergencies. Make sure that:

☐ Small objects are kept out of children's reach.
☐ Toy box has ventilation holes.
☐ If there is a lid, it is lightweight and removable and has a sliding door or panel or is a hinged lid with a support to hold it open.
☐ The crib mattress fits the side of the crib snugly and toys, blankets and pillows are removed from the crib.
☐ Drape and blind cords are wound up and not dangling.
☐ Drawstrings are no longer than 3 inches.

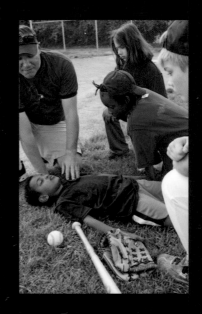

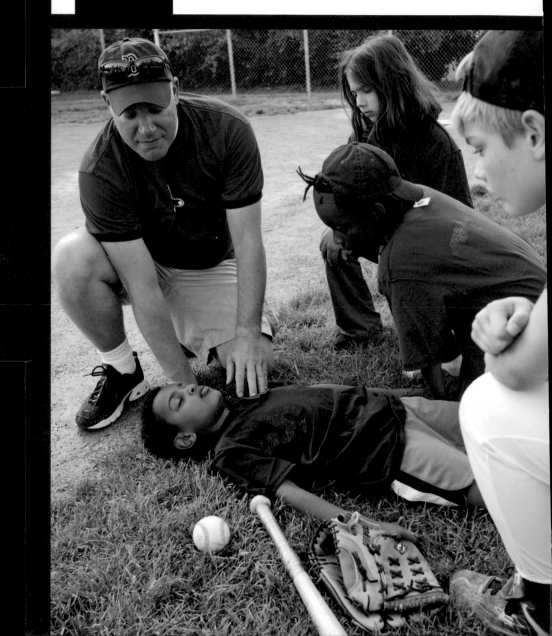

2

Emergency Action Steps

During a medical emergency, you may feel afraid, confused and unsure what to do. Above all, remain calm so you can think more clearly. Then follow the emergency action steps, CHECK—CALL—CARE, so you can respond effectively.

Check

Check the Scene for Safety

When an unusual noise, sight, odor or your child's appearance or behavior catches your attention and suggests something is wrong, your first reaction will likely be to investigate and try to help. But before rushing to help an ill or injured child, do a quick scan of the area. Make sure there is nothing that could hurt you before approaching the child. If it is not safe to approach the child, CALL or have someone else call 9-1-1 or the local emergency number to get help on its way as quickly as possible.

Also, look for any clues that may show what happened. For example, you might see a fallen ladder, broken glass, spilled medicine or a crumpled bicycle, which may suggest what kind of injuries or problems to look for.

IMPORTANT: If giving first aid care to a child or infant who is not your own, get permission from the child's parent or guardian, if one is present, before giving care. If the parent or guardian is not present, permission is implied in a life-threatening situation.

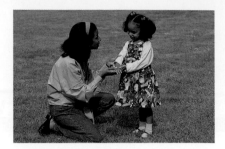

Check the Child

Once you are sure it is safe to approach, immediately check the ill or injured child to see if he is awake, breathing or bleeding. Tap or gently shake him (or, if an infant, you can flick the inside of his foot) and ask, "Are you ok?"

If he answers, moans or cries out, you will know he is conscious. Reassure him and try to find out what happened. If he doesn't respond, however, assume he is unconscious.

This is a life-threatening emergency, so call, or have someone else call, 9-1-1 or the local emergency number right away.

If a child or infant is unconscious, open the child's or infant's airway by tilting the head back and lifting up on the chin, and then check for signs of life (movement and normal breathing), then look for severe bleeding. Care for the conditions you find. See also Breathing Emergencies, page 52; Bleeding [Severe], page 65.

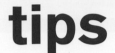

tips

Recognizing an Emergency

It is important that you know when a situation has become an emergency, and how to recognize life-threatening and nonlife-threatening emergencies so you can react properly and take care of your child.

An emergency is any situation where action is needed right away. Some emergencies involve calling 9-1-1 or the local emergency number, and some don't.

To recognize an emergency, use your senses and pay attention to:

- Unusual sights.
- Unusual noises (silence can also be an unusual "noise" with children).
- Unusual odors (or smells).
- Unusual appearances or behaviors.

These signals could mean that you need to take action quickly to protect yourself and the children.

Emergencies may also involve the weather, such as a flood or tornado, which requires immediate action to get you and your child to safety. Other emergencies that require you to take action include fires, explosions or violence. (See Chapter 5: How to Prepare for Any Emergency, page 105.)

First Aid Emergencies

A first aid emergency involves an injury or sudden illness. All first aid emergencies require your immediate action. Some involve calling 9-1-1 or the local emergency number; others do not. For example, a cut on your child's finger requires your prompt action, but not a call to 9-1-1; however, a child who is not breathing is experiencing a life-threatening emergency, requiring a call to 9-1-1 or the local emergency number.

Life-threatening emergencies are situations that could cause death quickly if you do not take immediate action. Learn more about how to respond to first aid emergencies by enrolling in a first aid and CPR course at your local Red Cross chapter (*www.redcross.org*).

IMPORTANT: The American Red Cross recommends that parents wear nonlatex, disposable gloves when caring for their child to prevent infection as well as use breathing barriers, such as resuscitation masks or face shields, when giving rescue breaths. However, parents should not delay providing care to their child if disposable gloves and breathing barriers are not available.

Call

Calling 9-1-1 or the local emergency number is often the most important thing you can do to help an ill or injured child. It's the fastest way to get medical help.

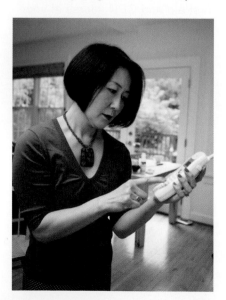

When to Call 9-1-1 or the Local Emergency Number

CALL 9-1-1 or the local emergency number and begin care if a child or infant:

- Is or becomes unconscious.
- Has difficulty breathing.
- Has skin or lips that appear blue, purple or gray.
- Is bleeding severely.
- Has neck stiffness or a rash with fever.
- Has a head injury with loss of consciousness, confusion and vomiting.
- Vomits blood or passes blood.
- Is unable to move or acts strangely.
- Has increasing or severe, persistent pain.
- Has a severe (critical) burn, particularly one involving the hands, groin or face.
- Has abdominal pain or pressure that does not go away.
- Has a seizure, severe headache or slurred speech.
- Appears to have been poisoned.
- Has neck or back injuries.
- Has a possible broken bone.
- Is a victim of electric shock.

Also be sure to CALL 9-1-1 or the local emergency number if the situation involves—

- Fire or explosion.
- Downed electric wires.

- Swiftly moving or rapidly rising water.
- Poisonous gas.
- Vehicle collisions.
- Children who cannot be moved easily.

How to Call 9-1-1 or the Local Emergency Number

When calling 9-1-1 or the local emergency number, stay calm and provide the following information:

- Your name
- The phone number from which you are calling
- What happened
- The exact location or address of the emergency (including intersections, landmarks, building name and/or apartment number)
- How many people are injured
- The condition of the injured
- What first aid is being given

After the call taker or dispatcher hangs up, continue to care for the child while waiting for emergency medical services (EMS) personnel to arrive.

IMPORTANT: Do not hang up until the call taker or dispatcher hangs up. The EMS call taker may be able to tell you what first aid to give until EMS arrives. If possible, have someone else make the call while you care for the child.

What to Do If You Are Alone

If you are the only person at the scene of a medical emergency, shout loudly for help. If no one arrives, you must decide whether to call 9-1-1 or the local emergency number first or give care before you call. Here are some guidelines to help you decide.

Call First. CALL 9-1-1 or the local emergency number **before** giving care for:

- A child about 12 years old or older who is unconscious.
- A child or an infant who suddenly collapses.
- An unconscious child or infant who you know has heart problems.

Care First. Give **2 minutes of care** before calling 9-1-1 or the local emergency number for:

- An unconscious child (younger than about age 12) whom you did not see collapse.
- Any victim of a drowning.

In most cases, you will **Care First** for a child or an infant who is unconscious because the cause is most likely a

tips

When to Call Your Pediatrician

Call your doctor instead of emergency services if your child is exhibiting:

- Vomiting and diarrhea that last for more than a few days or shows signs of dehydration, regardless of your child's age.
- A rash, especially if there is also a fever.
- Any cough or cold that does not get better in several days, or a cold that gets worse and is accompanied by a fever.
- Nasal congestion or cold symptoms, especially if your baby is 3 months or younger.
- Cuts that might need stitches.
- Limping or is unable to move an arm or leg.
- Ear pain with fever or that results in a child unable to sleep or eat, who vomits or has diarrhea, or who has ear infections that last longer than a day or if symptoms don't improve or get worse.
- Drainage from an ear.
- Diarrhea that doesn't go away.
- A sore throat or problems swallowing.
- Sharp or persistent pains in the abdomen or stomach.
- A fever (a temperature over 100.4° F) in infants younger than 3 months and a high fever (103° F) in children younger than 2 years of age.
- Fever and vomiting at the same time.
- Reflux, especially in infants, which could cause respiratory problems.
- Urinary tract infections.
- Rash or flu-like symptoms that may be related to a tick bite.
- Sunburn with blisters or a sunburn involving a large area.
- Finger injuries that include a deep cut, blood under the fingernail or if the finger looks like it might be broken.
- Minor head injuries if accompanied by changes in your child's condition or if your child vomits more than twice; cannot stop crying; has difficulty walking, talking or seeing; acts confused or abnormally; becomes drowsy or has trouble waking up; or has abnormal movements or seizures.
- Chest pain that is severe and lasts more than an hour, trouble breathing or is breathing fast.
- Headaches, if they occur more than once a week, are so severe that your child can't do normal activities, that wake your child up or occur in the early morning, that cause visual problems or a headache associated with vomiting, fever or a stiff neck.

breathing emergency, not a cardiac (heart) emergency. For a child or infant who has stopped breathing, you must get air into the child's lungs quickly to prevent the situation from becoming worse. For an unconscious adult or adolescent (about 12 years old or older), however, you will generally **Call First** because adults and adolescents are more likely to suffer from cardiac emergencies. In this case, the focus is on calling 9-1-1 or the local emergency number first to get EMS personnel with life-saving equipment, medications and emergency medical training on the scene as quickly as possible.

Care ⊚

Once you have checked the scene and the child and made a decision about calling 9-1-1 or the local emergency number, you may need to give care until EMS personnel arrive.

Go to Chapter 3: Life-Threatening First Aid Emergencies, page 41, and Chapter 4: First Aid Reference Guide, page 67, to learn how to respond to life-threatening emergencies and other first aid conditions.

Recovery Position

If you are alone and must leave a child for any reason—such as to call for help—or if the child is breathing normally but remains unconscious, place the child in a recovery position (on one side) (top photo). This will help keep the airway clear if the child vomits.

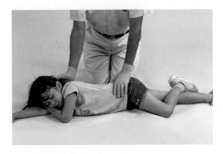

If you suspect a head, neck or back injury, move the child onto his or her side while keeping the head, neck and back in a straight line by placing the child in a modified High Arm In Endangered Spine (H.A.IN.E.S.) position (bottom photo).

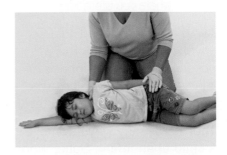

Emergency Moves

While giving care to an ill or injured child, you'll also need to decide if the child should be moved.

One of the most dangerous threats to a seriously injured child or infant is unnecessary movement. You should move an injured child or an infant **ONLY** in the following situations:

- When you are faced with immediate danger, such as fire.
- When you have to get to another person who may have a more serious injury or illness.
- When you need to move the child or infant to give proper care.

If you must move the child for one of these reasons, you must quickly decide how to move him. Carefully consider your safety and the safety of the child. To avoid hurting yourself or the child, use your legs, not your back, when you bend. Bend at the knees and hips and avoid twisting your body. Walk forward when possible, taking small steps and looking where you are going.

Avoid twisting or bending anyone who you think has a possible head, neck or back injury. Do not move a child who is too large to move comfortably.

There are many ways to move a child or an infant. Some work better in certain situations than in others. Review the following emergency moves to know what to do in case your child is injured and needs to be moved.

Walking Assist. To help a child who needs help walking to safety:

1. Place the child's arm around your shoulders or waist, depending on the child's size, and hold it in place with one hand.
2. Support the child with your other hand around the child's waist.
3. Move the child to safety.

Another person, if present, can support the child in the same way on the other side.

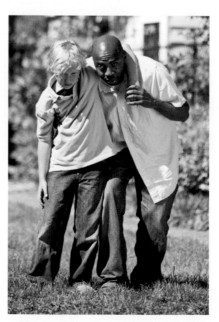

Two-Person Seat Carry. To carry a child who cannot walk and who you do not think has a head, neck or back injury:

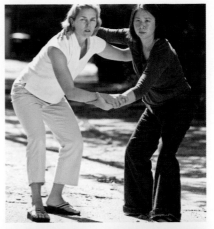

- Put one arm under the child's thighs and the other across the child's back, under his arms.
- Interlock your arms with another person's arms under the child's legs and across the child's back.
- Lift the child in the "seat" formed by your interlocked arms.
- Move the child to safety.

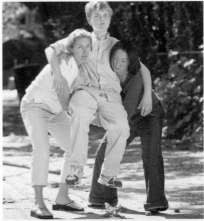

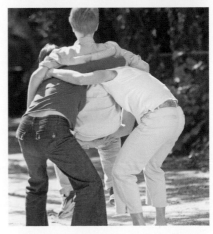

Clothes Drag. To move a child or an infant who may have a head, neck or back injury:

- Gather the child's or infant's clothing behind his neck.
- Pull the child or infant to safety.

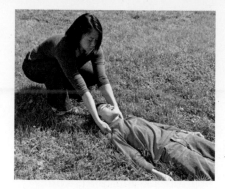

While moving the child or infant, cradle the head with his clothes and your hands.

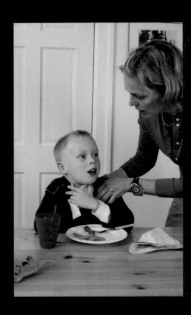

3

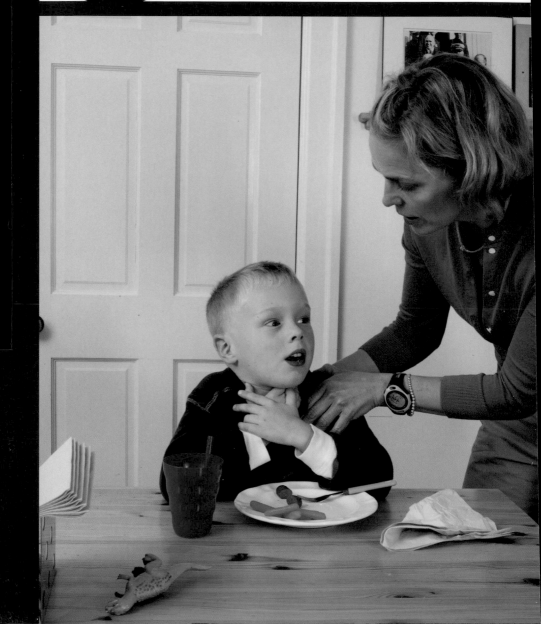

Life-Threatening
First Aid Emergencies

When a life-threatening emergency occurs with your child, you want to be able to react quickly and effectively. This chapter addresses the most severe life-threatening first aid emergencies and how to give appropriate care. Review this information *before* you need it, but it is not a substitute for training that you would receive in an American Red Cross course. The Red Cross *strongly* recommends that you take a course in cardiopulmonary resuscitation (CPR) and first aid to become better prepared to care for these life-threatening emergencies.

Breathing Emergencies

There are two types of breathing emergencies—respiratory distress (i.e., breathing is difficult) and respiratory arrest (i.e., breathing stops completely). It is especially important to recognize breathing emergencies in children (about age 12 or younger) and infants and to act before the heart stops beating. Seconds count when breathing stops. (See also Allergic Reaction, page 69; Asthma, page 70; Choking—Conscious Child, page 55; Choking—Conscious Infant, page 56; Choking—Unconscious Child or Infant, page 57; Rescue Breathing, page 58; and Drowning, page 83.)

What to Look For. Signs of a breathing emergency are when a child or infant:

- Is unable to relax or be still.
- Is upset or agitated.
- Is dizzy or sleepy.
- Has pale, blue or ashen (gray) skin color.
- Has blue lips or fingernails.
- Has unusually fast or slow breathing.
- Has noisy breathing including wheezing, gurgling or whistling.

0 minutes: **Breathing stops. Heart will soon stop beating.**

4–6 minutes: **Brain damage possible.**

6–10 minutes: **Brain damage likely.**

Over 10 minutes: **Irreversible brain damage certain.**

- Has hoarse crying or coughing in a way that sounds like barking.
- Grasps his throat.
- Cannot cough, cry, speak or breathe.
- Has a surprised, confused or panicked look, which may be accompanied by silence.
- Breathes so hard you can see the muscles between his ribs going in and out.
- Has pain in chest and/or back with breathing.

What to Do.
- CHECK the scene to make sure it is safe.
- Send someone to CALL 9-1-1 or the local emergency number.

If the child or infant is conscious:

- Have the child or infant rest in a comfortable position.
- CHECK and CARE for the conditions you find.
- If the child cannot cough, speak or breathe, give CARE for choking. (See Choking, page 54.)

If the child or infant is unconscious:

- Tilt the head back and lift the chin to open the airway.
  - Place one hand on your child's (A) or infant's (B) forehead and tilt the head back while pulling up on the bony part of the jaw to lift the chin with your other hand. This will open the airway.
- Look, listen and feel for signs of life (movement and normal breathing) for no more than 10 seconds.
- If the child or infant is unconscious but breathing normally, place in a recovery position and treat the conditions you find. (See Recovery Position, page 47.)

IMPORTANT: Do not confuse irregular, gasping or shallow breaths with normal breathing.

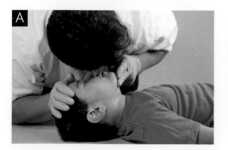

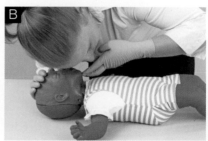

If the child or infant is NOT breathing, give 2 rescue breaths.

- Tilt the head and lift the chin, then pinch the nose shut.
- Make a seal over a child's mouth, (C) but seal over an infant's mouth *and* nose. (D) Be careful not to overextend the baby's neck when tilting the head back.
- Give 2 breaths, about 1 second each, making the child's or infant's chest clearly rise.

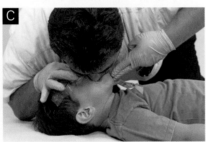

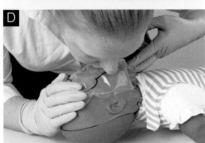

If the chest does NOT clearly rise, go to Choking—Unconscious Child and Infant, page 57.

If the chest clearly rises:

- If you are trained in how to feel for a pulse, then CHECK

for a pulse for no more than 10 seconds. (E, F)

- If you find a pulse, give rescue breathing. (See Rescue Breathing, page 58.)

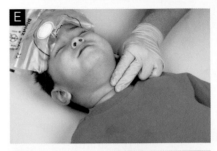

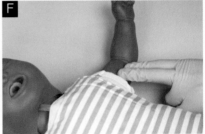

- If you are not trained in how to give rescue breathing or cannot feel a pulse or are not sure:
  - Give CPR or use an automated external defibrillator (AED) if one is immediately available and you are trained to do so. (See Cardiopulmonary Resuscitation, page 60; Automated External Defibrillator, page 64.)

Choking
To a young child, everything in the world exists to be put in the mouth. That's why young

children have such a high risk of choking. But even a 10-year-old can choke on a piece of candy. The following will show you what to do to clear a child's airway.

Choking—Conscious Child.

What to Look For. A child may be choking if he or she:

- Clutches the throat with one or both hands.
- Cannot cough, speak or breathe.
- Coughs weakly or is making high-pitched sounds.

What to Do.

- CHECK the scene and the child.
- Send someone to CALL 9-1-1 or the local emergency number.
- Give CARE.

If your child is coughing forcefully, encourage him to keep coughing. If he can't cough, speak or breathe:

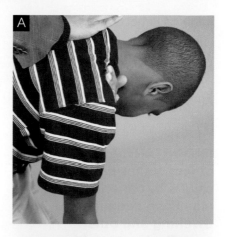

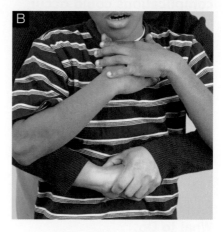

- Give 5 back blows with the heel of your hand between your child's shoulder blades. (A)
  - Lean your child forward, providing support by placing one of your arms diagonally across his chest to the far shoulder.
- Then give 5 quick, upward abdominal thrusts. (B) To do this:
  - Place the thumb side of your fist against the middle of your child's abdomen, just above the navel.
- Grab your fist with your other hand.
- Repeat the back blows and abdominal thrusts until:
  - The object is forced out and your child breathes or coughs forcefully on his own OR
- Your child becomes unconscious.

If the child becomes unconscious, CALL 9-1-1 or the local emergency number if you have not already done so and continue giving care. (See Choking—Unconscious Child and Infant, page 57.)

IMPORTANT: Even if an object comes out, your child's throat and airway may have been injured. Swelling and other complications could occur, so any child who has choked needs prompt medical care.

Choking—
Conscious Infant.
What to Look For. An infant may be choking if he or she:

- Cannot cough, cry or breathe.
- Coughs weakly or makes high-pitched sounds.

What to Do.
- CHECK the scene and the infant.
- Send someone to CALL 9-1-1 or the local emergency number.
- Give CARE.

If the infant is coughing forcefully, do not give back blows or chest thrusts. If the infant is unable to cough, cry or breathe:

- Give 5 firm back blows (between the shoulder blades) with the heel of your hand (A):
  - Place the infant face-up along your forearm.
  - Place your other hand on top of the infant, using your thumb and fingers to hold the jaw while sandwiching the infant between your forearms.
  - Turn the infant over so the infant is face-down on your forearm.
  - Lower your arm onto your thigh so the infant's head is lower than the chest.

IMPORTANT: Hold your infant's head and neck securely when giving back blows and chest thrusts.

If the airway is still blocked:

- Give 5 chest thrusts. (B)
  - Place the pads of 2 or 3 fingers just below an imaginary line between the nipples.
  - Compress the chest smoothly to a depth of about ½ to 1 inch.

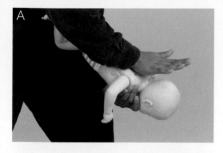

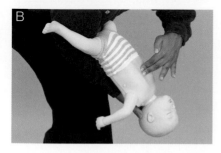

Repeat back blows and chest thrusts until:

- The object is forced out and the infant breathes or coughs forcefully on her own

OR

- The infant becomes unconscious.

IMPORTANT: If the infant becomes unconscious and you have not already done so, CALL 9-1-1 or the local emergency number IMMEDIATELY and give CARE for an unconscious choking victim. (See Choking–Unconscious Child and Infant, page 57.)

Choking—Unconscious Child and Infant.

What to Look For. The infant or child is not breathing and you are unable to make the chest clearly rise when giving rescue breaths.

What to Do.

- CHECK the scene and the child or infant. Tap the child's shoulder or flick the infant's foot and shout, "Are you okay?"
- If no response, CALL or send someone to call 9-1-1 or the local emergency number. If alone, give 2 minutes of CARE and then CALL 9-1-1 or the local emergency number.
- Try 2 rescue breaths:
  - Tilt the head and lift the chin, then pinch the nose shut.
  - Make a seal over a child's mouth, but seal over an infant's mouth *and* nose. Be careful not to overextend the baby's neck when tilting the head back.
  - Give 2 breaths, about 1 second each.

If the breaths don't go in:

- Retilt the head down and back to the open position (for an infant, do not tilt the head back as far).
- Try 2 more rescue breaths.

If his chest doesn't rise:

- Give 30 chest compressions.
  - For a child ages 1 to about age 12:
    - Place the heel of one hand on the center of the chest.
    - Place your other hand directly on top of your first hand. Try to keep your fingers off the chest by interlacing them or holding them upward. (A)
    - Position yourself so your shoulders are directly over your hands and compress the child's chest 30 times, pushing down fast and deep (about 1–½ inches).
  - For an infant under about age 1:
    - Place the pads of 2 or 3 fingers just below an imaginary line between the nipples.
    - Compress the chest smoothly 30 times to a depth of about ½ to 1 inch. (B)
- Open the mouth and look for an object. (C, D)
- If you can see the object, remove it with your finger. (E) (For an infant, use your small finger). (F)
- Try 2 rescue breaths. (G, H)

If the breaths still do not go in:

- Continue sets of 30 chest compressions, followed by looking for an object/removal and giving 2 rescue breaths until:
  - The child's or infant's chest clearly rises with rescue breaths.
  - The child or infant starts breathing.
  - EMS arrives.
  - Another trained responder takes over.
  - You are too exhausted to continue.
  - The scene becomes unsafe.

If your breaths go in:

- CHECK for signs of life (movement and normal breathing) for no more than 10 seconds.
- Give CARE based on the conditions you find.

Rescue Breathing
- Rescue breathing is a technique used to provide a nonbreathing child or infant with oxygen. Give rescue breathing only if you are trained to do so.

What to Look For.
- The child or infant is not breathing but has a pulse.

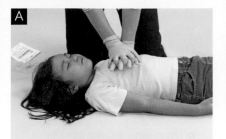

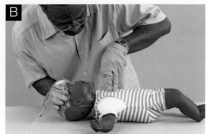

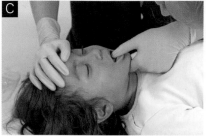

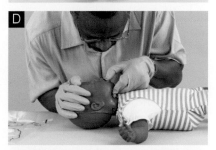

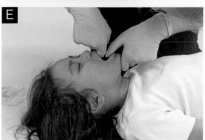

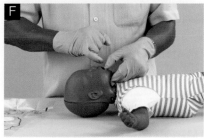

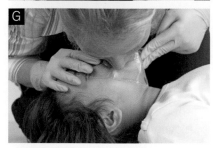

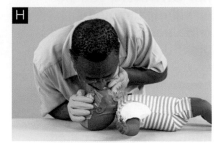

What to Do.

- CHECK the scene and your child or infant.
- CALL 9-1-1 or the local emergency number.
- Tilt the head back and lift the chin.

- Place one hand on your child's or infant's forehead and tilt the head back while pulling up on the bony part of the jaw to lift the chin with your other hand. This will open the airway.

- CHECK for signs of life (movement and normal breathing) for no more than 10 seconds.
- Give 2 rescue breaths.
  - Tilt the child's head and lift the chin, then pinch the nose shut.
  - Make a seal over a child's mouth, but seal over an infant's mouth *and* nose. Be careful not to overextend the baby's neck when tilting the head back.
- Give 1 rescue breath about every 3 seconds, making the child's or infant's chest clearly rise.
- After about 2 minutes, recheck signs of life and pulse for no more than 10 seconds. CARE for the conditions you find.

IMPORTANT: If you are unwilling, unable or untrained to give rescue breathing or full CPR (chest compressions and rescue breaths), give continuous chest compressions after 9-1-1 or the local emergency number has been called. Continue chest compressions until EMS arrives or you find an obvious sign of life. (See Continuous Chest Compressions, page 62.)

Continue giving CARE until:

- The scene becomes unsafe.
- You find an obvious sign of life such as normal breathing.
- An AED is ready to use.
- You are too exhausted to continue.
- Another trained responder arrives and takes over.

Cardiac (Heart) Emergencies

Children (ages 1 year to about 12 years) and infants seldom initially suffer a cardiac (heart) emergency. Instead, they suffer a breathing emergency, such as a severe asthma attack that leads to a cardiac emergency. Motor vehicle crashes, drowning, suffocation, poisoning, choking and smoke from fires are also all common causes of breathing emergencies that can develop into a cardiac emergency.

Cardiopulmonary Resuscitation (CPR)
What to Look For.
- The child or infant does not respond or is unconscious.
- There are no signs of life (no movement or normal breathing).

What to Do.
- CHECK the scene and your child or infant.
- CALL 9-1-1 or the local emergency number.
- Tilt the head back and lift the chin.

- Place one hand on your child's or infant's forehead and tilt the head back while pulling up on the bony part of the jaw to lift the chin with your other hand. This will open the airway.
- CHECK for signs of life (movement and normal breathing) for no more than 10 seconds.
- Give 2 rescue breaths.
  - Tilt the child's head and lift the chin, then pinch the nose shut.
  - Make a seal over a child's mouth, but seal over an infant's mouth *and* nose. Be careful not to overextend the baby's neck when tilting the head back.
- Give 2 rescue breaths, about 1 second each, making the child's or infant's chest clearly rise.
- Begin full CPR.

CPR for a Child (Ages 1 Year to About 12 Years).

- Place the heel of one hand on the center of your child's chest. (A)
- Place your other hand directly on top of your first hand. Try to keep your fingers off the chest by interlacing them or holding them upward.
- Position yourself so your shoulders are directly over your hands and compress the child's chest 30 times, pushing down fast and deep (B)

(about 1½ inches for a child).
- Give 2 rescue breaths. (C)

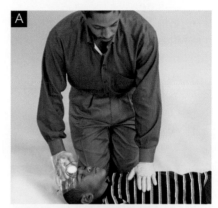

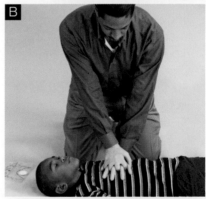

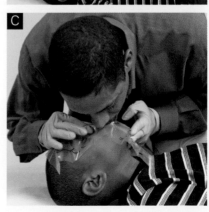

- Continue cycles of 30 chest compressions and 2 rescue breaths until:
  - The scene becomes unsafe.
  - You find an obvious sign of life such as movement or normal breathing.
  - An AED is ready to use.
  - You are too exhausted to continue.
  - Another trained responder arrives and takes over.

CPR for an Infant (Under Age 1)

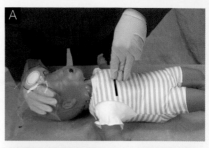

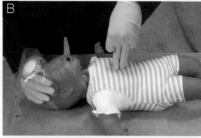

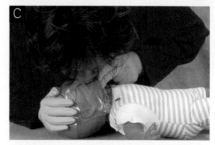

- Place the pads of 2 or 3 fingers just below an imaginary line between the nipples. (A)
- Compress the chest smoothly 30 times to a depth of about ½ to 1 inch. (B)
- Give 2 rescue breaths. (C)
- Continue cycles of 30 chest compressions and 2 rescue breaths until:
  - The scene becomes unsafe.
  - You find an obvious sign of life such as normal breathing.
  - You are too exhausted to continue.
  - Another trained responder arrives and takes over.

IMPORTANT: If you are unwilling, unable or untrained to give full CPR (with rescue breaths), give continuous chest compressions after calling 9-1-1 or the local emergency number. Continue chest compressions until emergency medical services arrives or you find an obvious sign of life.

Continuous Chest Compressions

Continuous chest compressions help keep a person's blood

circulating until help can arrive. They should be given when a person is unwilling, unable or untrained to give full CPR (chest compressions with rescue breaths).

What to Look For.
- The child or infant does not respond or is unconscious.
- There are no signs of life (no movement or normal breathing).

What to Do.
- CHECK the scene and the child or infant.
- CALL 9-1-1 or the local emergency number.
- Tilt your child's or infant's forehead back and lift the chin to open the airway.
- CHECK for signs of life (movement and normal breathing) for no more than 10 seconds.

For a child ages 1 year to about 12 years:

- Place the heel of one hand on the center of your child's chest.
- Place your other hand directly on top of your first hand. Try to keep your fingers off the chest by interlacing them or holding them upward.
- Position yourself so your shoulders are directly over your hands and compress the child's chest 30 times, pushing down fast and deep (about 1 ½ inches for a child).
- Continue chest compressions until the scene becomes unsafe, you find an obvious sign of life (such as movement or normal breathing), an AED is ready to use, you are too exhausted to continue or a trained responder arrives and takes over.

For an infant under age 1:

- Place the pads of 2 or 3 fingers just below an imaginary line between the nipples.
- Compress the chest smoothly 30 times to a depth of about ½ to 1 inch.
- Continue chest compressions until the scene becomes unsafe, you find an obvious sign of life (such as movement or normal breathing), an AED is ready to use, you are too exhausted to continue or a trained responder arrives and takes over.

IMPORTANT:

- **For a child about ages 1 year to about 12 years, compress the chest about 1½ inches.**
- **For an infant under age 1, use 2 or 3 fingers to compress the chest about ½ to 1 inch.**

Automated External Defibrillator (AED)

What to Look For. There are no signs of life.

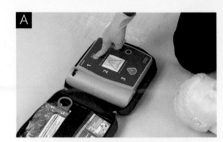

IMPORTANT: Continue CPR until the AED is ready to use. Minimize interruptions of chest compressions.

IMPORTANT: Use pediatric pads for children from birth to 8 years, or who weigh less than 55 pounds, if available. If pads on a child risk touching each other, put one on his front and one on his back. (F, G)

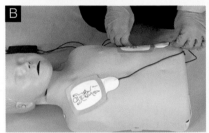

What to Do. If an AED is ready to use:

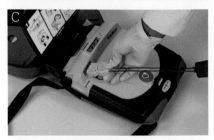

- Turn it on. (A)
- Wipe the child's chest dry.
- Attach the pads to bare chest. (B)
- Plug in the connector, if necessary. (C)
- Make sure no one, including you, is touching the child.
- Tell everyone to "STAND CLEAR." (D)
- Push the "analyze" button, if necessary, and let the AED analyze the child's heart rhythm.

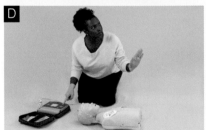

If the AED advises you to shock the child or infant:

- Make sure no one, including you, is touching the child or infant.

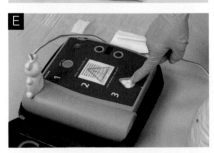

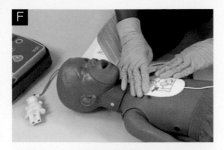

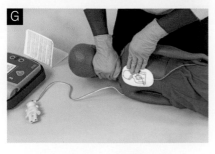

- Tell everyone to "STAND CLEAR."
- Push the "shock" button if necessary. (E)

After the shock is delivered:

- Give 5 cycles or about 2 minutes of CPR (30 chest compressions and 2 rescue breaths per cycle).
- Let the AED reanalyze the child's or infant's heart rhythm.
- If the AED says, "no shock advised," give 5 cycles, or about 2 minutes, of CPR.
- Follow the AED prompts.

Bleeding (Severe)

Any bleeding by a child can be frightening. But if you get frightened, you're only going to scare your child. So remain calm and assess the situation.

An open wound can be as minor as a scrape or as severe as a deep penetration. The amount of bleeding depends on where the wound occurred and how severe the injury is. If the bleeding stops quickly and there is very little blood, then it is considered minor bleeding. When minor bleeding occurs, see Minor Injuries (Cuts, Scrapes and Abrasions), page 95. Take the following steps when caring for a major wound.

Major Wounds
A major wound is one in which:

- The bleeding cannot be stopped.
- The wound shows muscle, bone or involves joints, hands, feet or the face.
- The wound is large or deep.
- Large or deeply embedded objects are in the wound.
- The wound was caused by a human or animal bite.
- Skin or body parts are partially or completely torn away.

IMPORTANT: CALL 9-1-1 or the local emergency number for any of these situations.

What to Do. If your child has suffered a major wound, remember CHECK–CALL–CARE:

- CHECK the scene and your child.
- Have someone CALL 9-1-1 or the local emergency number.
- Cover the wound with a sterile dressing and apply direct pressure. Avoid touching blood or body fluids by wearing disposable gloves or using a similar, clean barrier. (A)
- Cover the dressing with a bandage and apply direct pressure to the wound until the bleeding stops. (B)
- If bleeding continues and the wound soaks through the bandage, do not remove the bandage. Apply additional bandages on top of the others and apply more pressure.
- CHECK for feeling, warmth and color of the child's limb after applying the bandage.

IMPORTANT: Always wash your hands with soap and water immediately after giving CARE, even if you used disposable gloves.

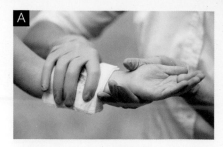

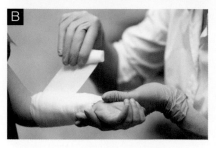

If the bleeding doesn't stop:

- Apply an additional dressing and bandage, applying more pressure.
- CALL 9-1-1 or the local emergency number if you have not already done so.
- CARE for shock. (See Shock, page 102.)

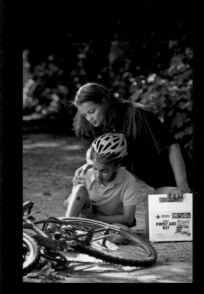

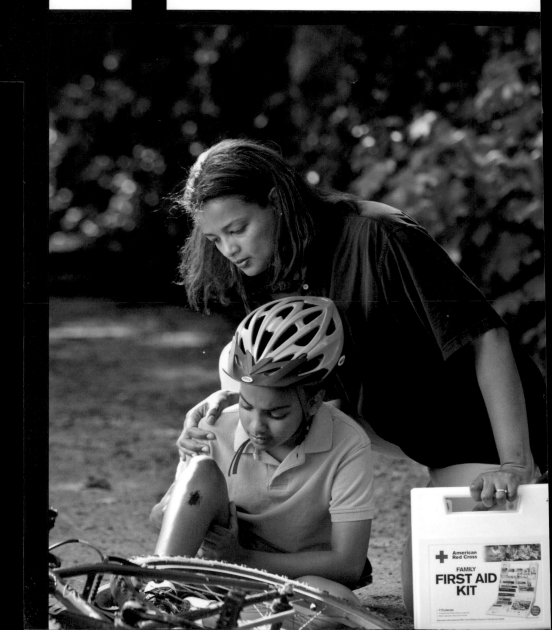

First Aid
Reference Guide

When your child is sick or injured, you need to know what to do. This section offers an overview of the most common illnesses and injuries that can occur in children. Review this information *before* you need it, but it is not a substitute for training that you would receive in an American Red Cross course. Contact your local Red Cross chapter to sign up for a first aid class so you can be prepared.

Abdominal Pain and Stomachaches

Spitting up, vomiting and stomachaches are common occurrences in infants and young children. Fortunately, most are not serious and usually go away on their own. If your child has a fever with stomach pain or vomiting, see your doctor. Related conditions include:

- **Appendicitis.** This condition, in which the appendix becomes infected, is relatively uncommon in infants. Symptoms include pain that starts in the center of the abdomen then moves down and over to the right lower side. The child may have a slight fever, loss of appetite and vomiting. CALL your doctor at once.

- **Colic.** This is a condition that typically occurs in infants age 3 months and younger. It may be caused by intestinal gas, food sensitivity or allergy or an immature nervous system. Your baby may cry inconsolably for several hours a day, typically in the late afternoon and early evening. Movement, including walking and driving in a car, can help, as can the sound from a vacuum in the next room or the clothes dryer. You also can hold your baby using certain techniques to help relieve gas pain. Consult with your doctor, who should diagnose colic after ruling out more serious medical conditions.

- **Constipation.** Infants are rarely constipated, but older children can become constipated, resulting in abdominal pain. You may need to add more high-fiber foods to their diet, such as whole-grain cereals, fruits and vegetables and increase the amount of water your child drinks. Do not give laxatives to children. If the constipation persists or abdominal pain occurs, see your doctor.

- **Emotional upset.** In children older than age 5, but sometimes even younger, a stomachache can signal some type of emotional upset or stress. In this situation, the pain tends to come and go over a week or so, and is not accompanied by other symptoms, such as vomiting or fever. Talk to your child to try to find out what's going on. If necessary, bring her in to see the doctor or another health care professional who can help her talk about what's bothering her.

- **Intestinal infection (*gastroenteritis*).** This is the most likely cause of stomach upset and typically includes vomiting and diarrhea. It is usually caused by a virus, which requires no treatment. Keep your child well hydrated with liquids, including commercially available oral rehydration solutions specifically designed for infants and children. If the symptoms persist for more than a few days, or if you think your child may be getting dehydrated, CALL your doctor immediately. Signs of dehydration include less frequent urination, crying without tears, dry mouth, dark-colored urine and reduced activity.
- **Lead poisoning.** If you live in a home built before 1977, when regulations prohibiting lead in paint went into effect, your child may have ingested lead. One symptom is abdominal pain. If you suspect lead poisoning, ask your doctor to test your child's blood lead levels.
- **Reflux.** Gastroesophageal reflux occurs during or after a meal when contents in the stomach "reflux," or back up into the esophagus, causing a burning feeling. Smaller meals; avoiding carbonated drinks, chocolate, caffeine and high-fat or spicy food; and elevating the head of your child's bed should help. In infants, this reflux could cause respiratory problems. Medications are available to help treat severe reflux, however. CALL your doctor.
- **Urinary tract infections.** These are more common in children younger than age 2 and in 3- to 5-year-old girls, but may occur in boys. Children may feel pain and burning when urinating, experience abdominal or back pain, have some bed-wetting or urinate more often than normal. In young children, symptoms may include fever and abdominal pain with vomiting and diarrhea. CALL your doctor.

Allergic Reaction

An allergic reaction occurs when the immune system over-responds after exposure to a substance. Some allergies for infants and children include bee stings, pollen, animals and some foods such as milk, nuts or shellfish. An allergic reaction can range from minor, such as a mild skin rash caused by contact with poison ivy or sneezing from pollen, to life threatening, such as when a swollen airway makes breathing difficult. If you notice an unusual inflammation or rash on a child's skin just after he has come into contact with a substance he is allergic to, the child may be having an allergic reaction. If minor allergic reactions become uncomfortable or prolonged, see your doctor.

Anaphylactic Shock

Anaphylactic shock (also known as anaphylaxis) is a life-threatening allergic reaction. Signs include:

* Trouble breathing.
* A tight feeling in the chest and throat.
* Swelling of the face, neck and tongue.
* A rash or hives.
* Dizziness or confusion.
* An allergic reaction, such as rash, hives and itching.
* Abdominal cramping, vomiting or diarrhea.

What to Do.

* CHECK the scene to make sure it is safe.
* CHECK your child carefully for swelling and breathing problems.
* CALL 9-1-1 or the local emergency number.

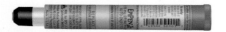

IMPORTANT: If a child uses a prescribed epinephrine auto-injector for severe allergic reactions, a parent should administer the injection as directed by their physician and the manufacturer's instructions as soon as symptoms begin.

Asthma

Asthma is a chronic respiratory illness. It can be controlled with medication, but sometimes an asthma attack can occur in which the airways swell, causing breathing difficulty. This can be very frightening to a young child (and to you!). Attacks can be triggered by infections, exercise, cold air, strong emotions, allergens or other irritants.

IMPORTANT: If your child suffers from asthma, follow your doctor's recommendations and reduce known allergens (i.e., allergy "triggers") in the environment as much as possible. Be sure your child takes anti-inflammatory medications as prescribed and carries an inhaler with quick-relief medication to relieve symptoms of a sudden attack.

Signs of an Asthma Attack

During a severe asthma attack, your child may exhibit the following:

- Difficulty breathing, shortness of breath
- Coughing or wheezing noises
- Rapid, shallow breathing
- Sweating
- Tightness in the chest
- Inability to talk without stopping for breath
- Fear or confusion

What to Do. Don't panic! Your calmness will help your child remain calm and ease breathing difficulties. Put your child in a comfortable position sitting up. Then:

- Loosen any tight clothing, especially around his neck and abdomen.
- Give him a dose of his "rescue" medication as prescribed and directed by your physician.
- CALL 9-1-1 or the local emergency number if his breathing difficulty does not improve in a few minutes, is severe, gets worse or if your child is not behaving normally.

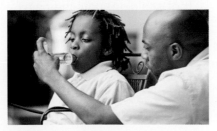

Back Injuries

See Head, Neck and Back Injuries, page 90.

Bites and Stings

Although the bite of a domestic or wild animal can cause infection, the most serious potential result is rabies. If not treated, rabies is fatal. Anyone bitten by an animal that might have rabies *must* receive prompt medical attention.

Insect bites and stings, while painful, are rarely fatal. However, if someone has a severe allergic reaction (see Allergic Reaction, page 69) to the bite or sting, it can result in a breathing emergency. (See Breathing Emergencies, page 52.) A child who has been bitten or stung will feel pain. Check for a bite mark or stinger and any swelling or bleeding.

Animal Bites

If your child has been bitten by an animal, look for a bite mark, bleeding, pain and swelling.

What to Do.

- Wash the wound with soap and water if the bleeding is minor.
- Control the bleeding.
- Apply triple antibiotic ointment if the child has no known allergies or sensitivities to the medication.

- Cover with a dressing.
- Get immediate medical attention if the wound bleeds severely (see Bleeding [Severe], page 65) or if you are unsure if the animal has rabies.
- CALL 9-1-1 or the local emergency number or contact animal control. **Never try to restrain or capture an animal yourself.**

IMPORTANT: Rabid animals may drool, appear partially paralyzed, act aggressively or behave in a strange way. Stay away!

Insect Stings
What to Do. If your child is stung by a bee or other insect:

- Remove the stinger. You can do this by scraping the stinger away with a flat surface, such as a credit card. Otherwise, carefully remove it with tweezers, being sure to grab the base of the stinger to avoid squeezing the venom sac.
- Wash the wound with soap and water.

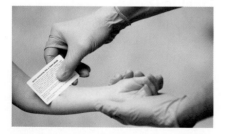

- Cover the wound with a dressing.
- Apply ice or a cold pack.
- Watch for signals of severe allergic reaction.
- CALL 9-1-1 or the local emergency number if there are signs of severe allergic reaction; otherwise, CALL your pediatrician.
- If your child displays signs of anaphylaxis, use an epinephrine auto-injector, if prescribed.

Marine-Life Stings
Nothing ruins a day at the beach quicker than a jellyfish sting. Signs your child has been stung include:

- Possible marks.
- Pain.
- Swelling.
- Possible allergic reaction. (See Allergic Reaction, page 69.)

What to Do.
- If your child has been stung by a jellyfish, soak the area in vinegar as soon as possible. Salt water also can be used to flush away any stinger cells.
- If you think it is a stingray, soak the area in hot water (not scalding) until the pain goes away.
- Clean and bandage the wound.
- CALL 9-1-1 or the local emergency number if your child develops an allergic reaction.

Snake Bites

Not all snakes are poisonous, but don't take any chances. If you see a bite mark, pain or swelling on your child, and a snake is in the immediate area, take action. Pay attention to color, head shape and markings on the snake so you can describe it to emergency medical personnel.

What to Do. If bitten by a pit viper (rattlesnake, copperhead, cottonmouth):

- CALL 9-1-1 or the local emergency number.
- Wash wound.
- Keep the bitten body part still and lower than your child's heart.

If bitten by an elapid snake (e.g., coral snake):

- Follow the above steps and apply an elastic roller bandage to fit snugly but not tight (you should be able to easily fit a finger under the bandage). (See Family First Aid Kit, page 107.)
- CHECK feeling, warmth and color of limb before and after applying bandage, to make sure the limb has not been wrapped too tightly.
- Begin wrapping the bandage at the point on the limb farthest from the heart.

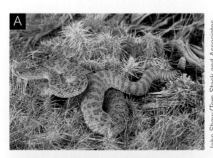
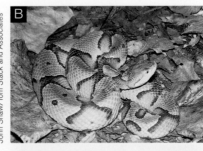
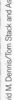
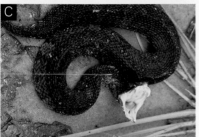
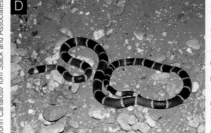

John Shaw/Tom Stack and Associates

David M. Dennis/Tom Stack and Associates

John Canalosi/Tom Stack and Associates

David M. Dennis/Tom Stack and Associates

A-Rattlesnake, B-Copperhead, C-Cottonmouth, D-Coral snake.

Spider Bites and Scorpion Stings

Signs of a spider bite or scorpion sting include:

- Bite mark.
- Swelling.
- Pain.
- Nausea and vomiting.
- Trouble breathing or swallowing. (See Allergic Reaction, page 69.)

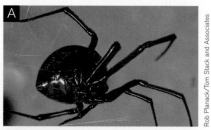

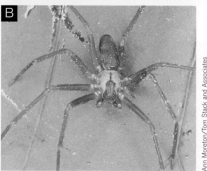

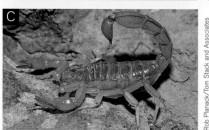

A-Black widow spider, B-Brown recluse spider, C-Scorpion.

What to Do. If your child has been bitten by a spider:

- Wash the wound.
- Cover with gauze.
- Apply ice or a cold pack.
- CALL 9-1-1 or the local emergency number if there are signs of severe allergic reaction or significant swelling.

Tick Bites and Lyme Disease

Children can get Lyme disease from the bite of an infected deer tick. This tick is much smaller than a dog tick—about the size of a poppy seed or the head of a pin. It is difficult to see and its bite is often painless, so your child may not even know she's been bitten.

A rash will start as a small red area at the site of the bite and may appear a few days or a few weeks after the bite. Other signs include:

- On fair skin—the center may be lighter in color and the outer edges red and raised (bull's-eye appearance).
- On dark skin—the area may look black and blue.
- Fever, headache, weakness.
- Flu-like joint and muscle pain.

What to Do. To remove the tick:

- Wear disposable gloves, then grasp the tick with fine-tipped, pointed, nonetched,

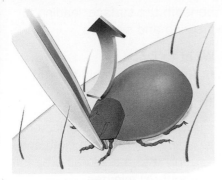

nonrasped tweezers close to the skin and pull slowly.
- DO NOT try to burn the tick off.
- DO NOT apply petroleum jelly or nail polish to the tick.
- If you cannot remove the tick, or if its mouth parts remain embedded, get medical care.

If you can remove the tick:

- Wash the bite area with soap and water.
- Apply antiseptic or triple antibiotic ointment, if available (if your child has no known allergies or sensitivities to the product).
- If rash or flu-like signals appear, CALL your health-care provider immediately.

Bleeding

Infants and children get scrapes and scratches frequently. Wounds and injuries bleed when blood vessels under the skin are torn or damaged.

Bleeding (Minor)

If the bleeding stops quickly and there is very little blood, it is considered minor bleeding.

What to Do.

- Control any bleeding (with direct pressure).
- Wash the wound with soap and warm water. If possible, rinse with clean running tap water for about 5 minutes to remove any visible dirt or debris.
- Apply triple antibiotic ointment if the child or infant has no known allergies or sensitivities to the medication.
- Cover the wound with a sterile bandage.

See Minor Injuries (Cuts, Scrapes and Abrasions), page 95.

Bleeding (Severe)

See Bleeding (Severe), page 65, in Chapter 3: Life-Threatening First Aid Emergencies.

Blisters

A "hot spot," or a tender area, that typically appears on the feet or hands is the early sign of a blister. Eventually, it becomes a raised area filled with clear fluid or, sometimes, blood. Blisters can be painful for children.

What to Do.
- CHECK the child or infant.
- Remove your child's shoe and sock (if the blister is on the foot).
- Cover any sore spots or closed blisters with thin, sterile gauze, then cover with a bandage. Have your child wear a different pair of shoes if the blister is on a foot.

Important: Don't puncture, drain or cut blisters that are not broken. This could cause infection.

If a blister is broken:

- Wash the skin with soap and water.
- Wipe the area with an antiseptic wipe.
- Apply a triple antibiotic ointment if the child or infant is not allergic or sensitive to the medication, cover with thin gauze and apply a bandage.

Breathing Emergencies
See Breathing Emergencies, page 52, in Chapter 3: Life-Threatening First Aid Emergencies.

Bruises and Swelling
Any time you bump yourself or bang into something, you can break delicate blood vessels beneath the surface, leading to bruising and swelling.

What to Do.
- Apply ice or a cold pack to help control pain and swelling.
- Fill a plastic bag with ice or wrap ice in a damp cloth and apply it to the injured area for about 20 minutes.
- Place a cloth, or a thin barrier such as a gauze pad, between the source of cold and the skin to prevent injury.
- Elevate the injured part to reduce swelling. DO NOT elevate if it causes more pain.

IMPORTANT: If continued icing is needed, remove the ice pack for 20 minutes, then replace it.

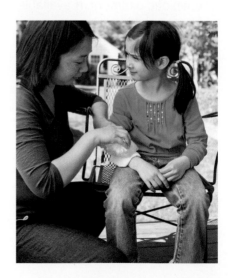

Burns

Critical burns can be life threatening, disfiguring and disabling, but the information below can help reduce the possibility of serious injury.

Always CALL 9-1-1 or the local emergency number for burns that:

- Cause trouble with breathing.
- Cover a large area or more than one body part.
- Involve the head, neck, hands, feet, genitals, mouth or nose.
- Involve a child younger than age 5 (unless the burn is very minor).
- Were caused by chemicals, explosions or electricity.

Recognize a deep (serious) burn:

- The skin is red and has blisters that may open and weep clear fluid.
- The area may appear brown or black.
- Pain can range from very painful to nearly painless.

Electrical Burns

To identify electrical burns, look for:

- Burn marks on the skin (entry and exit of current).
- Unconsciousness.
- Dazed, confused behavior.
- Breathing difficulty.
- Weak, irregular or absent pulse.

What to Do.

- CHECK the scene to make sure it is safe.
- CHECK your child or infant.
- Send someone to CALL 9-1-1 or the local emergency number.

IMPORTANT: DO NOT go near your child or infant until the power is turned off at its source, such as the main circuit breaker. Keep in mind that cordless and some other home telephones may not work without power. DO NOT go near downed power lines.

Be prepared to give CPR or use an AED. (See Cardiac [Heart] Emergencies, CPR–Child, page 61, or CPR–Infant, page 62.)

CARE for shock and thermal burns. (See Shock, page 102, and Heat [Thermal] Burns, page 78.)

Chemical Burns

Signs of a chemical burn include:

- Chemical on the skin.
- Swelling, red skin.
- Pain, burning or stinging sensation.

What to Do.

- CHECK the scene to make sure it is safe.
- CHECK your child or infant.
- Send someone to CALL 9-1-1 or the local emergency number.

For a dry chemical:

- Brush dry chemicals off your child's skin with a gloved hand before flushing with large amounts of cool water.
- Take care not to get any in your eyes or in your child's eyes.
- Use a gloved hand to remove jewelry and contaminated clothing that may trap chemicals against the skin or on which chemicals may have spilled.

For a wet chemical:

- Flush the affected areas with large amounts of cool running water for at least 20 minutes or until EMS personnel arrive.
- Always flush away from the body.

Heat (Thermal) Burns
What to Do.
- CHECK the scene to make sure it is safe.
- CHECK your child or infant.
- Stop the burning. Remove your child or infant from the source of the burn and put out the flames.
- Cool the burn. Use large amounts of cold running water until the pain recedes. Do not use ice to cool the burn.
- Cover the burn loosely with a sterile dressing and CARE for shock. (Go to Shock, page 102.)

- For a serious burn, CALL, or have someone else call, 9-1-1 or the local emergency number.

Radiation (Sunburns)
Signs of sunburn include:

- Red, painful skin with possible blisters.
- Swelling.

What to Do. If your child is sunburned:

- Cool the burn by holding it under cool running water or by fanning the area.
- Protect unbroken blisters with loose bandages and keep broken blisters clean to prevent infection.
- Protect her from further damage by keeping her out of the sun and having her wear sunscreen when she's outside.
- If there are blisters or the burn involves a large area, CALL your doctor.

Stop, Drop and Roll
Be sure everyone in your family knows what to do if their clothes ever catch on fire.

- Stop; do not run.
- Drop to the ground.
- Roll on the ground to put out the flames. Cover your mouth, nose, eyes and face with your hands while doing this to protect your airway.

Chest Pain

Sudden chest pain in a child is generally caused by a bad cough, which can lead to sore muscles in the chest wall, or the aftermath of a too-vigorous workout. It also can be caused by respiratory problems such as asthma or infections. Heart disease is rarely ever the cause of chest pain in children. Treat sore muscles with acetaminophen or ibuprofen, following directions for your child's weight and age. A warm compress or heating pad can also help. The pain should go away within a few days.

CALL your doctor IMMEDIATELY if:

- The pain is severe and lasts for more than an hour.
- Your child has trouble breathing or is breathing fast.
- Your child is acting very sick.

Choking—Conscious Child

See Choking—Conscious Child, page 55, in Chapter 3: Life-Threatening First Aid Emergencies.

Choking—Conscious Infant

See Choking—Conscious Infant, page 56, in Chapter 3: Life-Threatening First Aid Emergencies.

Choking—Unconscious Child or Infant

See Choking—Unconscious Child·or Infant, page 57, in Chapter 3: Life-Threatening First Aid Emergencies.

Common Cold, Nasal Congestion, Croup and the Flu

Expect your child to catch numerous colds throughout childhood. You'll also be dealing with what might seem like an inordinate number of runny noses and coughs, not to mention the flu. Don't worry; it's just childhood!

Colds and Nasal Congestion What to Do. Infants and children usually don't need any special care for colds or nasal congestion, which are caused by viruses. However, if your baby is 3 months old or younger, CALL your doctor at the first sign of illness.

IMPORTANT: There is no medication for a cold. Antibiotics are not effective against colds. They will only help if a bacterial infection develops.

Other important things to know about colds:

- Do not give cold remedies to your infant or young child (age 3 and younger) without first checking with your health-care provider.
- You can help relieve your child's nasal congestion by using saline drops and a cool-mist humidifier while your child is sleeping.
- If your infant is having trouble nursing because of a stuffy nose, use a bulb syringe and saline drops to clear out her nose before feeding. Use of a cool-mist humidifier can also help relieve her congestion by keeping the mucous loose.
- Make sure your child washes her hands often to avoid passing on the virus to others in the household. And make sure you and anyone else taking care of her also wash their hands frequently.

Croup

Croup is an inflammation of the voice box and windpipe. It results in a barking cough, hoarseness and noisy breathing and is usually caused by a virus.

What to Do. If the coughing occurs in the middle of the night, fill the bathroom with warm, steamy air from the shower and sit in the room with your child until her breathing eases. Then use a cool-mist humidifier in her bedroom to moisturize the air and make it easier for her to breathe.

CALL the doctor or 9-1-1 or the local emergency number if:

- She makes a whistling sound that gets louder with each breath.
- She's unable to talk.
- She is struggling to breathe.
- She is blue or pale.

Flu

Like colds, the flu is caused by a virus, so antibiotics will not be effective.

What to Do. To help lessen your child's discomfort:

- Give acetaminophen or ibuprofen for fever and muscle aches.
- Have your child rest.
- Give extra fluids.
- Use a cool-mist humidifier to ease breathing.

IMPORTANT: Never give aspirin to a child who has a cold, the flu or is suspected of having the flu. Aspirin has been linked to a dangerous condition called Reye's syndrome in children with the flu.

To protect your child against the flu next year, consult with your doctor or a medical professional about when to get a flu vaccine. Flu vaccines are recommended for all children age 6 months and older with serious health problems and for all healthy children ages 2 through 17 years.

Convulsions and Seizures

High fevers can cause seizures or convulsions in young children, but seizures can also occur because of a condition known as epilepsy. These seizures are usually controllable with medication; however, even when infants and children are on medication, seizures can sometimes still occur.

What to Do. If your child has a seizure, immediately do the following:

- Lay him on the floor or bed away from hard or sharp objects.
- Turn his head to the side so any saliva or vomit can drain from his mouth.
- Don't put anything in his mouth. He won't swallow his tongue but could bite down on your finger or other objects in his mouth, breaking his teeth or injuring you.
- CALL your health-care provider when the seizure ends.

CALL 9-1-1 or the local emergency number immediately if:

- Your child has never had a seizure before.
- A seizure lasts longer than 5 minutes or is repeated.
- A seizure is followed by a quick rise in the child's temperature.
- Your child does not regain consciousness.
- Your child is diabetic or injured.
- Any life-threatening condition is found.

Diabetic Emergency

If your child has diabetes, she can become ill because there is too much or too little sugar in her blood. Signs include:

- Light-headedness, dizziness, confusion or weakness.
- Irregular breathing.
- Irregular pulse.
- Feeling or looking ill.
- Changes in her level of consciousness.

What to Do.
- CHECK the scene to make sure it is safe.
- CHECK the child, including her blood sugar level.

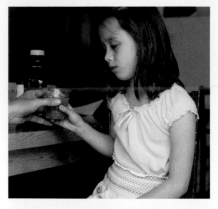

dehydration and is more likely to do so in young children. CALL your health-care provider if diarrhea persists for more than a few days or if your child:

- Hasn't had a wet diaper in 3 or more hours or, if older, has not had any urine output for more than 6 hours.
- Has a high fever.
- Has bloody or black stools.
- Is unusually sleepy, drowsy, unresponsive or irritable.
- Cries without tears or has a dry mouth.
- Has a sunken appearance to her abdomen, eyes or cheeks; or, in a very young infant, has a sunken soft spot at the top of her head.
- Has skin that remains "tented" if pinched and released.

Otherwise:

- If your infant will not tolerate her normal feedings or if a child is drinking less fluid than normal, add a commercially available oral rehydration solution specifically designed for infants and children.
- Do not give over-the-counter anti-diarrhea medications to children younger than age 2, and use with the guidance of your pediatrician in older children.

- If she is conscious and if you determine her blood sugar is low or if you can't check her blood sugar level and she can safely swallow food or fluids, give sugar (fruit juices, nondiet soft drinks, table sugar).
- If she isn't feeling better about 5 minutes after giving her the snack, CALL 9-1-1 or the local emergency number.

If the child is unconscious:

- DO NOT give her anything to eat or drink.
- Send someone to CALL 9-1-1 or the local emergency number.
- CHECK the child, then CARE for the conditions you find.

Diarrhea

Diarrhea, or loose stools, often accompanies an infection in children. However, it can lead to

- Maintain the same diet with your child; just try to limit sugar and artificial sweeteners. In addition, encourage your child to eat items like bananas, rice, applesauce and toast.

Drowning

What to Do. Drowning is a life-threatening emergency.

- Send someone to CALL 9-1-1 or the local emergency number.
- Attempt to rescue your child by reaching or throwing an object that floats to him.

IMPORTANT: DO NOT ATTEMPT A SWIMMING RESCUE UNLESS YOU HAVE PROPER EQUIPMENT AND ARE TRAINED TO DO SO.

Once your child is out of the water:

- Tilt his head back, lift his chin and CHECK for signs of life.

If he is breathing:

- Keep the airway open and monitor breathing.
- Make sure someone has called 9-1-1 or the local emergency number.

If he is not breathing:

- Give 2 rescue breaths. (See Breathing Emergencies, page 52.)

- If you are not trained to give rescue breaths, you should begin continuous chest compressions. (See Continuous Chest Compressions, page 62.)

If the breaths go in:

- Give CPR if you are trained to do so. (See Cardiopulmonary Resuscitation [CPR], page 60.) If not, give continuous chest compressions. (See Continuous Chest Compressions, page 62.)

If the breaths do not go in:

- Retilt your child's head and try 2 breaths again. (See Unconscious Choking—Child and Infant, page 57.)

Ear Injuries and Infections
Ear Injuries

Your child could get an injury to her ear in many ways, including falling off her bike or getting hit by the ball during volleyball. Other injuries could occur if a pierced earring catches on something and tears away from the ear. The eardrum can also be injured if your child is hit in the head, puts a foreign body into her ear or experiences sudden pressure changes, such as those caused by an explosion or a deep-water dive.

Signs of an eardrum injury include:

- Loss of hearing.
- Loss of balance.
- Inner ear pain.
- Bleeding from inside the ear.

If this occurs, CALL your health-care provider.

What to Do. If a foreign object such as dirt, an insect or cotton becomes stuck in the ear canal:

- If you can see and grasp the object, remove it with your fingers or tweezers. Do not try to remove any object by using a pin, toothpick or a similar sharp item. You could force the object farther back or puncture the eardrum.
- If you have trouble removing the object, try pulling down on the earlobe, tilting your child's head to the side and shaking or gently striking the head on the affected side.
- If you cannot easily remove the object, take your child to your health-care provider.

IMPORTANT: If your child has a serious head injury, blood or other fluid may be in the ear canal or may be draining from the ear. Do not attempt to stop this drainage with direct pressure. Instead, just cover the ear lightly with a sterile dressing. CALL 9-1-1 or the local emergency number.

Ear Infections

Your child may have many symptoms during an ear infection. Talk with your health-care provider about the best way to treat your child's symptoms, which include:

- Pain—the most common symptom of an ear infection is pain. While older children can tell you that their ears hurt, younger children may only cry or be irritable.
- Loss of appetite.
- Trouble sleeping.
- Fever.
- Ear drainage.
- Trouble hearing.

What to Do.

- If your child's signs and symptoms last longer than a day, CALL your health-care provider.
- Treat pain symptoms with ibuprofen or acetaminophen.
- In children younger than age 2, watch for sleeplessness and irritability during or after an upper respiratory infection, such as a cold.
- CALL your child's health-care provider if you see a discharge of blood or pus from the ear. This could indicate a ruptured eardrum.

- If your child has been diagnosed with an ear infection, CALL your child's health-care provider if your child's signs and symptoms don't improve or they get worse.

Embedded Object

If your child has an embedded object in him, he will be in pain and there likely will be some bleeding.

What to Do.

- CHECK the scene to make sure it is safe.
- Send someone to CALL 9-1-1 or the local emergency number.
- **DO NOT REMOVE THE OBJECT.**
- Place bulky dressings around the object to support it in place so it can't do any additional damage.
- Use a roller bandage to secure the dressing in place.

Eye Injuries and Infections

Injuries to the eye can involve the bone and soft tissue surrounding the eye or the eyeball. Blunt objects, like a fist or a baseball, may injure the eye area, or a smaller object may penetrate the eyeball. Injuries that penetrate the eyeball are very serious and can cause blindness.

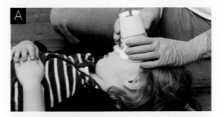

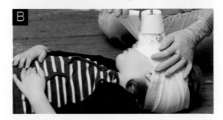

What to Do. If an object is in your child's eye, don't attempt to remove it. Instead:

- Put the child on her back.
- Put a sterile dressing around the object and stabilize it as best you can. You can stabilize it by placing a paper cup around the object to support it. (A)
- Bandage loosely and don't put any pressure on the injured eye or eyeball. (B)
- Seek immediate medical attention.

Dirt in the Eye

Foreign bodies, such as dirt, sand or slivers of wood or metal, that get in the eye can be quite painful and, left untreated, could cause significant damage. If your child has something in his eye, even light may irritate it.

What to Do. Follow these instructions to clear out the eye:

- Tell your child to blink several times. This creates more tears in an attempt to naturally flush the object out of the eye.
- If that doesn't work, try gently flushing the eye with water with a dropper or cup.
- If the object remains, seek medical care.

Conjunctivitis

Conjunctivitis (i.e., "pink eye") is a common childhood eye infection. Symptoms include redness in the white of the eye and the inside of the lower lid. You need to see your health-care provider as soon as possible for a diagnosis and medication in cases of bacterial infection.

Fever

Infants and children get numerous infections and illnesses throughout childhood, many resulting in fever. Fever itself is not an illness but a sign that the body's immune system is working to fight infection.

Infants with fever can:

- Be upset or fussy, with frequent crying.
- Be unusually quiet.
- Feel warm or hot.

- Breathe rapidly and have a rapid heart rate.
- Stop eating or sleeping normally.

IMPORTANT: CALL your health-care provider for infants younger than 3 months with any fever (temperature over 100.4° F) and children under 2 years old with a high fever (103° F).

Older children with fever can:

- Feel hot to the touch.
- Complain of being cold or chilled and body aches.
- Have a headache.
- Have trouble sleeping or sleep more than usual.
- Appear drowsy.
- Have no appetite.

What to Do. Once you confirm your child has a fever by taking her temperature:

- Make her as comfortable as possible and have her rest.

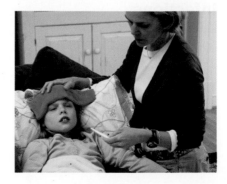

- Be sure she's not overdressed or under too many blankets. All she needs is a single layer of clothing and a light blanket.
- Encourage her to drink clear fluids such as water, juice or chicken soup to prevent dehydration.
- Give acetaminophen or ibuprofen for the fever.
- Closely watch your child for signs of life-threatening conditions, such as unconsciousness or trouble breathing, and CALL 9-1-1 or the local emergency number if necessary.

IMPORTANT: Do not give the child aspirin. For a child, taking aspirin can result in an extremely serious medical condition called Reye's syndrome.

High Fever
In a young child, even a minor infection can result in a rather high fever, which is often defined as a temperature above 103° F. Prolonged or excessively high fever can result in seizures. (See Convulsions and Seizures, page 81.)

What to Do. If your child has a high fever:

- Gently cool her.

- Remove excessive clothing or blankets and sponge the child with lukewarm water.
- CALL a physician at once if your child is younger than 2 years old. You should CALL your physician for any fever over 100.4° F in a child younger than 3 months.

Meningitis
Meningitis occurs when the tissues that cover the brain and spinal cord become inflamed due to either a virus or bacteria. The bacterial form, which is less common than the viral form, is the most serious. Symptoms of meningitis include fever, irritability, loss of appetite and sleepiness. Older children may complain of a stiff neck, back pain or a headache.

What to Do. See your health-care provider immediately to determine whether it is bacterial meningitis, which requires prompt treatment with antibiotics. Ask your doctor if your child should begin taking an antibiotic as a preventative if she has been exposed to someone else with bacterial meningitis.

If the illness is viral, there is no treatment, just supportive care for the fever and pain with acetaminophen or ibuprofen.

- The headache causes visual problems.
- Vomiting, fever or stiff neck accompany the headache.

Head, Neck and Back Injuries

You should suspect a serious head, neck or back injury if your child or infant:

- Was involved in a motor vehicle crash.
- Was injured as a result of a fall from a height greater than his own height.
- Says or indicates that his head, neck or back hurts.
- Has tingling, weakness or complains of loss of feeling in his arms or legs.
- Is not fully alert.
- Staggers when trying to walk.
- Appears weak.
- Loses all or part of movement in a body part.
- Has unusual bumps or depressions on his head, neck or back.
- Has blood or other fluids in his ears or nose.
- Has heavy external bleeding of his head, neck or back.
- Has seizures.
- Has trouble breathing or seeing as a result of the injury.
- Has nausea or vomiting.

- Has a headache that won't go away.
- Has loss of balance.
- Has bruising of the head, especially around the eyes and behind the ears.

What to Do.

- CHECK the scene to make sure it is safe.
- CHECK your child or infant.
- CALL 9-1-1 or the local emergency number.

If your child or infant is conscious—

- Keep the child or infant from moving.
- Place your hands on both sides of his head, keeping it in the position you found it.

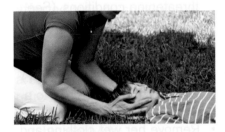

- If the head is sharply turned to one side, DO NOT move it. Support the head in the position you found it.

If your child or infant is unconscious—

- Carefully tilt his head back and lift his chin to open his airway. CHECK for signs of life (movement and normal breathing) for no more than 10 seconds. CARE for the conditions you find. (See also Cardiopulmonary Resuscitation [CPR], page 60; Automated External Defibrillator [AED], page 64.)

Minor Head Injuries (Bumps and Bruises)

Children frequently fall and bump their heads. If your child is alert and responds to you, it probably is just a minor head injury and usually no tests or X-rays are needed. He may cry from pain or fright. Most of the time, all he needs is a cuddle and kiss, but you may want to apply a cold compress for 20 minutes to reduce any swelling, then watch him closely for the first 24 hours. If he does well through the observation period, there should be no long-lasting problems. Remember, most head injuries are mild.

If there are any changes in your child's condition or if he experiences any of the following, CALL your pediatrician:

- Vomits more than twice
- Cannot stop crying
- Looks sicker
- Has difficulty walking, talking or seeing

- Acts confused or abnormally
- Becomes drowsy or you have trouble waking him
- Has abnormal movements or seizures or any behaviors that worry you

Scalp Injuries

Even minor cuts or lacerations to a child's scalp can bleed heavily because the scalp contains so many blood vessels. When checking a child with a head injury, look for swollen or bruised areas, but do not put direct pressure on any area that is swollen, depressed or soft.

What to Do. If your child has an open wound on her scalp:

- Control the bleeding with direct pressure.
- Apply several dressings and hold them in place with your hand.
- Press gently at first because the skull may be fractured. If you feel a depression, spongy area or bone fragments, do not put direct pressure on the wound. Instead, try to control bleeding with pressure on the area *around* the wound.
- Secure the dressings with a roller bandage or triangular bandage. (See Family First Aid Kit, page 107.)

- CALL 9-1-1 or the local emergency number if you are unsure about the extent of the injury or if there are any signs of a serious head injury as described above. EMS personnel will be better able to evaluate the injury.

See also Muscle, Bone and Joint Injuries, page 96.

Concussion

A concussion is a temporary impairment of brain function caused by a blow to the head and is considered a brain injury. Any concussion should be taken seriously. Signals of concussion include memory loss, concentration problems or confusion, nausea or vomiting, blurred vision or sensitivity to light, headache, speech difficulty, fatigue and coordination problems. Loss of consciousness may or may not occur with a concussion.

What to Do. If you suspect your child has suffered a concussion, CALL 9-1-1 or the local emergency number. If the blow occurred during a sporting event, don't let him return to the event until after seeing a medical professional.

Cheek Injury

An injury to the cheek usually involves only soft tissue. The most important thing is to control bleeding on the outside, inside or both sides of the cheek. Your child may swallow blood if there is bleeding inside the cheek, which could cause nausea or vomiting, complicating the situation.

What to Do. To control the bleeding:

- Place several dressings, folded or rolled, inside the mouth, against the cheek.
- Ask your child to hold the dressings in place, or you hold them with your hand.
- If there is external bleeding, place the dressings on the outside of the cheek and apply direct pressure.
- If an object passes completely through her cheek and becomes embedded, and you cannot control the bleeding with the object in place, remove the object to control the bleeding and keep the airway clear. You can remove the object by pulling it out in the same direction it entered.

IMPORTANT: This is the only exception to the general rule not to remove embedded objects from the body. An embedded object in the cheek cannot be easily

stabilized, makes control of bleeding more difficult and may become dislodged and obstruct the airway.

- Once the object is removed, fold or roll several dressings and place them inside your child's mouth. Also apply dressings to the outside of her cheek, being careful not to obstruct the airway.
- Sit her up leaning slightly forward so blood doesn't drain into her throat.
- As with any serious bleeding or embedded object, CALL 9-1-1 or the local emergency number.

Jaw Injury

Injuries serious enough to fracture or dislocate the jaw can also cause other head or neck injuries.

What to Do.
- CALL 9-1-1 or the local emergency number.
- Be sure to maintain an open airway.
- Also check inside the child's mouth for bleeding and control bleeding as you would for other head injuries, and minimize any movement of the head, neck or back.

Heat-Related Emergencies

Children can easily become overheated when playing outside in hot weather. Know what signs to look for if your child experiences a heat-related emergency.

Heat Cramps

Your child may get heat cramps, which are painful muscle spasms, usually in the legs and abdomen.

What to Do. If your child has heat cramps:

- Move her to a cool place.
- Give her small amounts of cool water to drink.
- Lightly stretch and gently massage the cramped area.
- DO NOT give salt tablets.
- Watch her carefully for signs of heat exhaustion or heat stroke.

Heat Exhaustion

Signs of heat exhaustion include:

- Cool, moist, pale, ashen (gray) or flushed skin color.
- Headache, nausea, dizziness.
- Weakness or exhaustion.
- Heavy sweating.

What to Do. If your child has heat exhaustion:

- Move her to a cool place.
- Loosen tight or remove perspiration-soaked clothing.
- Apply cool, wet cloths to her skin or mist with cool water.
- Fan her.

- If she is conscious, give her small amounts of cool water to drink.

If she doesn't improve quickly, refuses water, vomits, loses consciousness or shows signs of heat stroke, send someone to CALL 9-1-1 or the local emergency number. Then provide care for heat stroke. Otherwise, CALL your doctor.

Heat Stroke

Signs of heat stroke include:

- Red, hot, dry or moist skin.
- Changes in the child's level of consciousness.
- Rapid, weak pulse.
- Rapid, shallow breathing.
- Vomiting.

What to Do. Heat stroke is LIFE THREATENING! Send someone to CALL 9-1-1 or the local emergency number.

- Move your child or infant to a cool place and place him on his side in case he vomits.
- Loosen tight or remove perspiration-soaked clothing.
- Cool him by placing wet cloths on his skin or mist him with cool water. You can also place ice or cold packs on his wrists, ankles, groin, neck and armpits.
- Fan him.

- If he is conscious, give him small amounts of cool water to drink.

If your child or infant becomes unconscious, be prepared to give CPR, if necessary. (See CPR–Child, page 61; CPR–Infant, page 62.)

Infection (Wounds)

A wound has become infected if you see any of the following:

- Pus or cloudy fluid draining from the wound
- A pimple or yellow crust forming on the wound
- A scab that is getting larger
- Increasing redness around the wound
- A red streak spreading from the wound toward the heart

The wound may also be infected if:

- It has become extremely tender.
- The pain or swelling has increased 48 hours after the wound occurred.
- The lymph node draining that area of skin becomes large and tender.
- Your child develops a fever (temperature over 100.4° F).
- The wound hasn't healed within 10 days of the injury.

What to Do. If any of these occur, see your health-care

professional. Your child may need antibiotics or other medical care. Things you can do on your own include:

- For open wounds, soak the wounded area in warm water or put a warm, wet cloth over the wound for 20 minutes, three times a day. Use a warm saltwater solution with 2 teaspoons table salt per quart of water to remove all pus and loose scabs.
- For closed wounds, apply a heating pad or warm, moist washcloth to the reddened area for 20 minutes, three times a day.
- Give acetaminophen or ibuprofen for fever over 102° F or for wound pain.

Staph Infections

Staph infections are caused by common bacteria that live on the skin. But if the skin is broken through a scrape or other abrasion, the bacteria can get into your child's blood system, possibly causing a serious infection.

Staph infections on the skin look like a pimple or boil and can be red, swollen, painful or have pus or other drainage.

What to Do. If you suspect your child has a staph infection,

see your health-care provider. This is particularly important because some staph bacteria have become resistant to common antibiotics used to treat them.

The best way to avoid a staph infection is by reminding children to:

- Keep wounds covered.
- Wash their hands often with soap and water.
- Refrain from sharing personal items like clothing and towels.

Minor Cuts, Scrapes and Abrasions

What to Do. For cuts, scrapes and abrasions:

- CHECK the scene and your child or infant.
- Use a sterile gauze pad to apply direct pressure to control bleeding.
- Wash the wound with soap and water. Rinse for 5 minutes with clean, running tap water if possible.
- Apply a triple antibiotic ointment if your child has no known allergies or sensitivities to the medication.
- Cover the wound with a sterile dressing and bandage.
- Watch for signs of infection. (See Infection [Wound], page 94.)

IMPORTANT: Always wash your hands with soap and water immediately before and after giving CARE for minor injuries. Use an alcohol-based hand sanitizer if proper hand washing is not possible.

Mouth Pain and Injuries
Tooth (Knocked Out)

If your child has a tooth or teeth knocked out, remain calm. Reassure her that you're going to help.

What to Do. If she is conscious and able to cooperate:

- Rinse out her mouth with cold tap water, if available.
- Place a rolled sterile dressing in the space left by the tooth and ask her to bite down. This helps stop the bleeding.
- Save any knocked-out teeth. Place them in milk, if possible, or cool water.

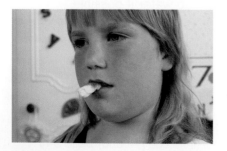

Pick the tooth up by the crown (white part), not the root.
- Take her to the dentist immediately.

Loose Tooth
What to Do.
- If the tooth is loose, check to see if it is chipped or cracked. Make sure no pieces are embedded in the lips, tongue or gums.
- Take your child to the dentist. The tooth may need to be stabilized or filed down.

Muscle, Bone and Joint Injuries

If your child is unable to move or use a body part, he may have a muscle, bone or joint injury. Examine the child for the following:

- Pain or discomfort.
- Bones or joints that do not look normal.
- Bruising or swelling.
- Pieces of bone that are sticking out of a wound.
- Bones that grate or were heard to snap or pop at the time of the injury.
- An injured area that is cold and numb.

Get medical care if the injury appears serious (e.g., if you suspect a fracture, there is an obvious deformity, severe pain, swelling or the child is unable to move a body part). CALL 9-1-1 or the local emergency number if you cannot transport your child safely.

What to Do. If you suspect a muscle, bone or joint injury, CARE for it by following RICE:

- **R**est—Avoid movement of the injured area.
- **I**mmobilize—Stabilize the injured area in the position found.
- **C**old—Apply ice to the injured area for 20-minute periods to control pain and swelling. Place a thin barrier between ice and bare skin. If continued icing is needed, remove the pack for 20 minutes, then replace it.
- **E**levate—Elevate the injured arm or leg ONLY if it does not cause more pain.

Splinting

Splinting is a method used to keep an injured body part from moving. It can also help reduce pain, making your child more comfortable.

- Since moving an injured body part can cause more harm, splint only if the child must be moved or transported and if you can do so without causing him more pain and discomfort.

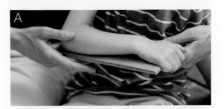

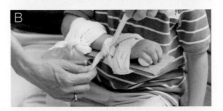

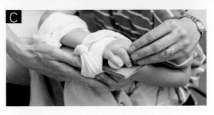

- Splint an injury in the position you find it. (A)
- Splint the joints above and below an injured bone.
- Splint the bones above and below an injured joint. (B)
- CHECK for feeling, warmth and color of the skin below the site of injury both before and after splinting. (C)
- If the injury appears serious, or your child cannot be safely transported, CALL 9-1-1 or the local emergency number.

What to Do. For a leg injury:

- CHECK the scene and the child.
- Immobilize the injured leg by binding it to the uninjured leg with a triangular bandage.

For fractured ribs:

- CHECK the scene and the child.
- Place a pillow or folded blanket between the injured ribs and the arm.
- Bind the arm to the body to help support the injured area.

For ankle and foot injuries:

- CHECK the scene and the child.
- Immobilize the ankle and foot by using a soft splint—a pillow or blanket.
- Do not remove the child's shoe.

For hand and finger injuries:

- CHECK the scene and the child.
- If you suspect that the finger is broken or dislocated, tape the injured finger to a finger next to it.

Nosebleeds

A blow from a blunt object (including a fist), high blood pressure, changes in altitude or dry air can cause nosebleeds.

What to Do. In most cases, you can control bleeding by having your child sit with his head slightly forward while pinching his nostrils together for 10 minutes.

Other methods of controlling bleeding include applying an ice pack to the bridge of the nose or putting pressure on the upper lip just beneath the nose. Keep your child leaning slightly forward so blood doesn't drain into his throat, which could lead to nausea and vomiting.

Seek additional medical care if the nosebleed continues after you try these techniques.

If your child loses consciousness, place him on his side to allow blood to drain from his nose and mouth. CALL 9-1-1 or the local emergency number immediately.

Poisoning

A poison is any substance that causes injury, illness or death if it enters the body.

Common causes of poisoning in infants and children include:

- Pain medications and cough and cold remedies.
- Topical medicines and gastrointestinal medications.
- Accidental ingestion of any medications belonging to an adult.
- Cleaning substance.
- Cosmetics and personal care products.
- Vitamins.
- Food products.
- Bites and stings.
- Plants.

Signs that your child may have been poisoned include:

- Seeing your child put something into his mouth or touch a poison before you can stop him.
- Burns around the lips or tongue, or on the skin.
- Open or spilled containers, open medicine cabinet, overturned or damaged plant.
- Trouble breathing, headache or dizziness.
- Nausea, vomiting, diarrhea.
- Chest or abdominal pain.
- Sweating, changes in consciousness, seizures.
- Unusual odors or smoke.

What to Do. If you suspect your child has been poisoned:

- CHECK the scene and look for any open containers, plants or bottles.
- If necessary, move him to safety, away from the source of the poison.
- CHECK your child.

IMPORTANT: DO NOT give your child anything to eat or drink unless directed to do so by the Poison Control Center or EMS.

If your child is conscious and is behaving normally with no breathing difficulties:

- Try to find out the type of poison, how much was taken and when it was taken.

- CALL the Poison Control Center hotline at (800)-222-1222 and follow their instructions.

If your child is unconscious, if his level of consciousness changes, or if you find another life-threatening problem:

- CALL 9-1-1 or the local emergency number.
- CARE for any life-threatening conditions, if found.
- Put the child on his side in case he vomits. If he does vomit, save a sample if you don't know what poison was involved so it can be identified at the hospital.
- Bring the item the child took or the bottle/container it came in to the hospital.

Household Chemicals
What to Do. For poisoning with dry chemicals on the skin:

- Brush off dry chemicals with gloved hand.
- Flush the area thoroughly with large amounts of cool water.
- Take care not to get any in your eyes or in the eyes of others.
- Remove jewelry and contaminated clothing that may trap chemicals against the skin or on which chemicals may have spilled.

If poisons such as wet chemicals get on the skin:

- Flush the affected area with large amounts of cool water for at least 20 minutes. Always flush away from the body.
- Have someone CALL 9-1-1 or the local emergency number.
- Keep flushing with cool water until EMS arrives.

Alcohol Poisoning

Signs of alcohol poisoning include:

- Confusion, stupor.
- Vomiting.
- Seizures.
- Slow or irregular breathing.
- Blue-tinged skin or pale skin.
- Low body temperature (hypothermia).
- Unconsciousness ("passing out").

What to Do. A child suffering from alcohol poisoning needs immediate attention.

- If unconscious, CALL 9-1-1 or the local emergency number.
- If conscious, CALL the National Poison Control Center hotline at (800)-222-1222 and follow their instructions.

- Do not try to make the child vomit; her gag reflex may be impaired and she could choke on or inhale her vomit.

Poisonous Plants

What to Do. If your child came in contact with poisonous plants, such as poison ivy (A), poison sumac (B) or poison oak (C):

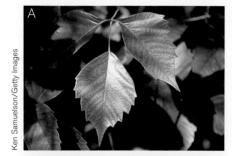

Ken Samuelson/Getty Images

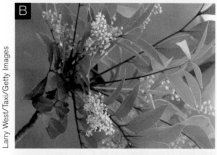

Larry West/Taxi/Getty Images

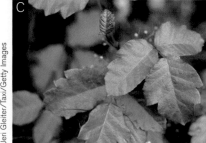

Jeri Gleiter/Taxi/Getty Images

- Immediately wash the affected area thoroughly with soap and water.
- If a rash or open sores develop, apply a paste of baking soda and water several times a day to reduce discomfort.
- Apply lotions such as calamine, which may help soothe the area, and hydrocortisone cream to control inflammation and itching.
- If the condition gets worse or affects large areas of the body or face, see a health-care provider.
- Wash all clothing exposed to plant oils.

Rashes

Infants and young children have very sensitive skin, prone to developing various rashes. Here's what you can do to help.

Heat Rash

Heat rash is a red or pink rash that forms on skin covered by clothing. It is most common with infants and looks like red dots or small pimples.

What to Do.

- Remove or loosen clothing to cool down your child.
- Move her to a cool location.
- Cool the area with wet washcloths or a cool bath and let the skin air dry.

If the area is still irritated, use calamine lotion or a hydrocortisone cream if your child is not sensitive or allergic to the cream. Avoid ointments or other lotions; they can irritate your child's skin.

Diaper Rash

When skin is wet for too long, it begins to break down, and when wet skin is rubbed, it becomes more damaged. Moisture from a dirty diaper can harm your child's skin, making it more irritated. This can cause a diaper rash to develop.

What to Do. Diaper rash in babies can generally be treated with a thick layer of over-the-counter diaper cream containing zinc oxide or petroleum jelly. These ointments create a barrier between the child's delicate skin and the urine or feces.

To prevent diaper rashes and help them heal:

- Keep the area as dry as possible by changing wet or soiled diapers immediately.
- Clean the area with water and a soft washcloth. Avoid wipes that can dry your child's skin.
- Pat dry, or let air dry.
- Keep the diaper loose so wet and soiled parts don't rub against skin.

See your health-care provider if the rash:

- Develops blisters or pus-filled sores.
- Does not go away within 2 to 3 days.
- Gets worse.

Eczema

Eczema is a skin condition marked by dry, red itchy skin. There are two types: "atopic dermatitis" and "contact dermatitis."

Atopic dermatitis is often seen in children with allergies or a family history of allergies, although it doesn't necessarily mean the child is allergic to something. The reddish rash may be itchy and scaly, and may ooze some pus or liquid.

Contact dermatitis results from irritation to a certain substance or fabric. Bubble baths, soaps, certain foods or medicines, even a child's own saliva can lead to contact dermatitis. This form of eczema doesn't itch as much as atopic dermatitis, and usually disappears once the child is no longer in contact with the offending material.

What to Do. To prevent and treat it:

- Keep the skin moist with moisturizing creams and ointments and avoid long, hot baths, which dry the skin.

- Avoid harsh or irritating clothing.
- If the rash is oozing or itching a lot, put tepid compresses on the area.

If the rash continues and is causing your child discomfort, fever, or if the rash spreads or shows evidence of infection, see your health-care provider. You may need a prescription cream or ointment. If the rash is suspected to be related to allergies, your doctor will refer you to a pediatric dermatologist or allergist for testing.

Seizures

See Convulsions and Seizures, page 81.

Shock

Shock can occur when a child has been injured. Shock is a medical description of a state of severe illness or injury, not an emotional response. Signs of shock include:

- Restlessness or irritability.
- Drowsiness, confusion or loss of consciousness.
- Nausea or vomiting.
- Rapid breathing and pulse.
- Pale or gray, cool, moist skin.
- Blue tinge to lips and fingernails.

What to Do. If your child is going into shock:

- CHECK the scene to make sure it is safe.
- CHECK your child.
- Send someone to CALL 9-1-1 or the local emergency number.
- Continue to closely watch your child's airway and breathing.
- Control any external bleeding.
- Keep her from getting chilled or overheated.
- Raise her legs about 12 inches if you do not think she has a head, neck or back injury or broken bones in her hips or legs. If you are unsure, keep her lying flat.
- Do not give her anything to eat or drink.
- Comfort and reassure her until EMS personnel arrive and take over.

Sprains (Joint Injury) and Strains (Muscle Injury)

See Muscle, Bone and Joint Injuries, page 96.

Stomachache

See Abdominal Pain, page 68.

Sunburn

See Burns, page 77.

Swallowed Objects

Given that infants and young children like to put everything in their mouths, it's not surprising that occasionally they will swallow something, like coins, small toys and other small objects. Most swallowed objects do not cause any symptoms and may pass out of the body on their own. Some objects may cause a child or infant to immediately choke and vomit. Depending on the type of item, such as a toy, there may be some pain or bleeding in the back of the throat.

If your child starts to choke, the following symptoms may occur:

- Drooling.
- Vomiting.
- Painful swallowing.
- Pain in chest or throat.
- Gagging.

A child may have no obvious symptoms or may exhibit:

- Refusal to eat (in infants).
- Weight loss and malnutrition.
- Vomiting blood.
- Blood in stool.
- Severe chest infection.

What to Do.
- If your child is choking, follow the steps recommend for choking in Choking, page 55.
- If your child is not choking but is experiencing any of the symptoms previously listed, take your child to your health-care provider immediately.

Vomiting

Vomiting can be frightening for a young child, but it's rarely a serious problem. However, it can lead to dehydration and is more likely to do so in young children. CALL your health-care provider if vomiting persists for more than a few days or if your child:

- Hasn't had a wet diaper in 3 or more hours or, if older, has not had any urine output for more than 6 hours.
- Has a high fever.
- Has bloody or black stools.
- Is unusually sleepy, drowsy, unresponsive or irritable.
- Cries without tears or has a dry mouth.
- Has a sunken appearance to her abdomen, eyes or cheeks; or, in a very young infant, has a sunken soft spot at the top of her head.
- Has skin that remains in place if pinched and released.

What to Do. If your infant or very young child is vomiting, lay him on his side so he doesn't swallow or inhale the vomit. If your child is vomiting and not replacing lost liquids, or can't retain liquids, he needs to see a health-care professional.

Also:

- Halt solid foods for 24 hours during an illness involving vomiting and replace with clear fluids, such as water, popsicles, gelatin water or an oral rehydration solution specifically designed for infants and children.
- Introduce liquids slowly. For instance, wait 2 to 3 hours after a vomiting episode to offer your child some cool water. Offer 1 to 2 ounces every half hour, four times. Then alternate 2 ounces of rehydration solution with 2 ounces of water every 2 hours.
- After 12 to 24 hours with no vomiting, gradually reintroduce your child's normal diet.

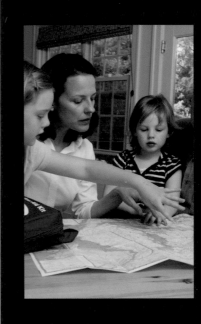

5

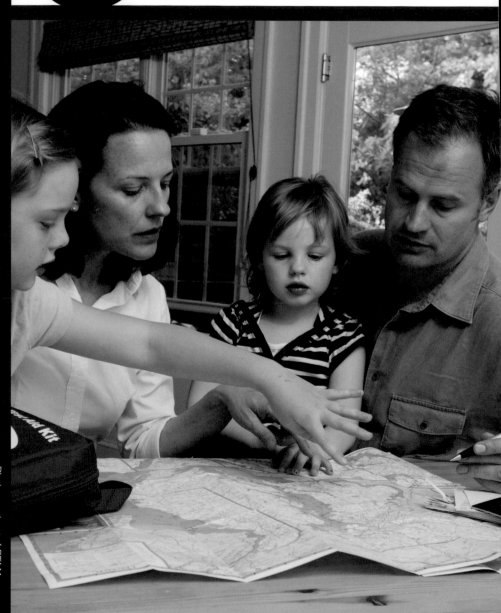

Know How to Prepare for Any Emergency

Parents and families need to know how to be prepared for an emergency, such as a serious injury or home fire. Other emergencies, whether a natural disaster like an earthquake or a flood or a human-caused disaster, such as a chemical spill or terrorist event, could also happen where you live. Be prepared so you can help your children and the other members of your family get through an unexpected emergency with a minimum of problems.

In this chapter you will learn about three key preparedness action steps you can take to provide you and your family with the peace of mind that comes from knowing how to Be Red Cross Ready:

- Get a kit.
- Make a plan.
- Be informed.

Get a Kit

Part of being Red Cross Ready involves having a well-stocked first aid kit in your home and in each vehicle. Store your first aid kit in an accessible location out of reach of young children. However, also make sure that older children know how to use the kit and where it is stored. You can purchase a family first aid kit at *www.redcross.org* or you can assemble your own using the Family First Aid Kit Checklist on page 107.

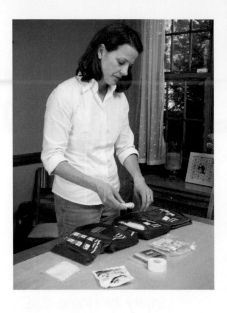

First Aid Kit: Dos and Don'ts

Antiseptic wipes. Use only for toddlers and older children, not on infants.

Instant cold compresses. When using an instant cold compress from your first aid kit, be very careful with infants. Their thinner skin and lower levels of fat could lead to hypothermia. Never apply a cold compress directly to the skin; always put a cloth or bandage between the compress and the child's skin. Do not use the compress for longer than 20 minutes at a time.

Digital thermometer. To use, place a clean thermometer cover over the tip, then place under the child's tongue and hold in place until it beeps. If using rectally, put some petroleum jelly on the end and, holding the child's anus open slightly, gently slide it in about an inch or less.

Tweezers. If you use tweezers to remove slivers in a child's skin, be very careful. If you can't get the sliver out, don't keep trying; bring your child to a medical professional. And don't use tweezers on an infant.

Family First Aid Kit Checklist

Item	Quantity	Suggested Use
Absorbent compress	2	Protect open wounds
Adhesive bandages (assorted sizes)	25	Protect open wounds
Adhesive tape (cloth) 1"	10 yards	Secure bandages or splints
Alcohol-based hand sanitizer	4 packets	Hand hygiene
Antiseptic wipe packets	5	Wound cleaning/germ killer
Aspirin (chewable) 81 mg	2	Heart attack symptoms in an adult.* Aspirin should not be given to children and infants.
Blanket (space blanket)	1	Maintain body temperature
CPR breathing barrier (w/one-way valve)	1	Protection from body fluids
First aid instruction booklet	1	
Gloves (large), disposable, nonlatex	2 pair	Prevent body fluid contact
Hydrocortisone ointment packets (approx 1 g ea.)	2	External rash treatment
Instant cold compress	1	Control swelling
Roller bandage 3" (individually wrapped)	1	Secure wound dressing
Roller bandage 4" (individually wrapped)	1	Secure wound dressing
Scissors	1	Cut tape, cloth or bandages
Sterile gauze pad 3" x 3"	5	Control external bleeding
Sterile gauze pad 4" x 4"	5	Control external bleeding
Thermometer, digital, oral (non-mercury/nonglass)	1	Take temperatures orally
Thermometer, digital, rectal (non-mercury/nonglass)	1	Take temperatures rectally
Triangular bandage	2	Sling or binder/splinting
Triple antibiotic ointment packets	5	Anti-infection
Tweezers	1	Remove splinters or ticks

*NOTE: Aspirin may be given only to adults if medically appropriate, but you must not delay calling 9-1-1 or the local emergency number during medical emergencies.

Disaster Supplies and Emergency Preparedness Kit

Having disaster supplies stored at home can help you and your family stay safe and fed in case basic services, such as water, gas, electricity or telephone, are suddenly cut off or normal supply chains are broken. It's a good idea to have enough food and water supplies to last 2 weeks or more at home in case you have to be on your own following a severe storm or power outage, or during a flu pandemic.

An emergency preparedness kit is also critical in case you have to evacuate your neighborhood,

workplace or school. Your emergency preparedness kit should contain at least 3 days of emergency supplies for each person and pet in your family. Collect the supplies in an easy-to-carry container like a duffle bag or plastic storage box so you can take it with you, if necessary.

An easy way to start your kit is to contact your local Red Cross chapter. You can also order an emergency preparedness kit online at *www.redcross.org.* Whether you decide to purchase a kit or build your own, make sure it includes the following items and check it every 6 months to replace expired items and ensure the clothing still fits your children and is still appropriate for the weather.

Keep Your Emergency Preparedness Kit Handy

Keep your emergency preparedness kit somewhere easy to get to. In other words, don't store it in the attic or away from your home. And keep a smaller version of the kit in each of your vehicles. This could be very important if you become stranded or are unable to return home during an emergency.

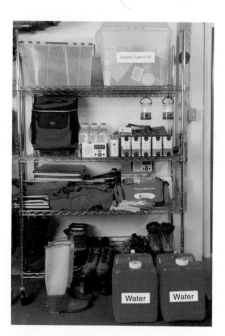

Emergency Preparedness Kit Checklist

Item	Quantity	Suggested Use
*Battery-powered or hand-crank flashlight (2 D-cell or equivalent [3 volt])	1	Provide light
*Battery-powered or hand-crank radio with instructions and extra batteries	1	Source for news and safety
Clothing and bedding—A change of clothes for everyone, including sturdy shoes, gloves and a sleeping bag or blanket		
Comfort items for children, such as toys and books		To occupy children during stressful situations
Contact information—A current list of family phone numbers and e-mail addresses, including someone out of the area who may be easier to reach if local phone lines are out of service or overloaded. Include pet-friendly hotels.	1	Communication link between family members
Duct tape (2" x 90')	1 roll	Seal plastic sheeting
Emergency blanket (Reflective, approximately 4.5' x 7')	1	Retain body heat (also first aid care for shock and hypothermia)
Emergency preparedness booklet		Information source
Extra pair of eyeglasses, contact lenses and solution		
*Food (Non-perishable, high-protein items, such as energy bars, ready-to-eat soup, peanut butter, etc. Stock foods that do not require refrigeration, preparation or cooking and little or no water.) Ensure that you have child-appropriate food for all of your children. Food Bars (60 percent total of protein and carbohydrates)	Minimum of 3-day supply	Source of nourishment
Gloves (work, leather or similar)	2 pair	Protect hands
Infant supplies (baby formula, diapers, bottles)		

* NOTE: Items with an asterisk (*) should be gathered first if you build a kit.

Emergency Preparedness Kit Checklist (*Continued*)

Item	Quantity	Suggested Use
Kitchen accessories and cooking utensils	as needed	Preparing and serving food
Map of area	1	Mark an evacuation route
*Medications (prescription and non-prescription)		In case local supply chains are cut off
Moist Towelettes (Individually wrapped)	6	Clean body or hands
Money (Cash)		ATMs and credit cards won't work if the power is out
*Personal documents (Copies of personal documents, including social security or other identification cards, insurance policies, birth certificates, passports, medical and immunization records and emergency information forms for all children with special health-care needs, etc.)	Varies, depending on need	In case your family has to evacuate immediately
Pet supplies (For each pet, include food, water, collar, leash, cage or carrier, litter box or plastic bags, tags, medications and vaccination information.)	Varies, depending on need	Keep animals safe and healthy
Plastic sheeting or heavy-duty garbage bags	1	Cover openings to "seal the room" during shelter-in-place
Rain poncho	1 for every family member	Protect clothing from rain/snow
Sanitary supplies (Bucket with tight-fitting lid, plastic bags, toilet paper, towelettes, feminine supplies, personal hygiene items, bleach, etc.)		Prevent spread of bacteria if indoor plumbing fails
Surgical and N95 breathing mask (NIOSH-42 CFR particles Part 84 certified)	1	Protect lungs from dust
Tools (Wrench to turn off gas, if necessary; manual can opener; screwdriver; hammer; pliers; knife)	1 each	Miscellaneous uses when necessary
*Water/water containers (At least 1 gallon per person per day, for drinking and sanitation)	At least a 3-day supply	Hydrate the body, sanitation
Whistle (Plastic, "pea less")	1	Help rescuers locate you

* NOTE: Items with an asterisk (*) should be gathered first if you build a kit.

Make a Plan

Everyone in your household should have a written plan describing what they should do and where they should go if a family emergency or regional disaster occurs. Also, make sure your children's teachers and caregivers have a copy of the plan, in case they need to reach you in an emergency.

The first step in creating such a plan is to talk about what types of emergencies may occur in your geographic area. When discussing these possibilities with your children, it's important to teach them without frightening them. Explain that a disaster is an event that could hurt people, and that sometimes nature provides "too much of a good thing," like rain, snow or wind.

Reassure your children that, although disasters can happen, there are often warnings and that even if there isn't, having a plan and an emergency preparedness kit can help keep everyone safer.

Important things to teach your children (depending on their age) include:

- How to call for help (9-1-1 or the local emergency number).
- When to call for help.
- Whom to call if they become separated from you.
- How and when to turn off utilities such as electricity, water and gas.
- Where emergency information, equipment and supplies are kept.

Every member of your family should have a responsibility in the event of an emergency so that you can work as a team. For instance, a younger child can help collect items, while an older child can leave a note with information about where the family has gone and when you left. Designate alternates for each job in case someone is absent.

It is also important that you consider how you will react if a family member is away for a long period of time. For instance, if someone in your family is deployed in the military, or travels frequently for work, how will you prepare on your own without them to help you?

Write It Down

Any emergency plan must be *written* down. After all, you could be anywhere when a disaster strikes—at work, at school or in the car. It's a good idea to keep a copy of the plan with you at all times, in a drawer at work, in

tips

Make Plans with Daycare Providers and Schools for Disasters and Emergencies

A disaster or emergency can occur at any time—including when your child is at daycare or in school. Make sure you know what your childcare provider's or your child's school's plans are for disasters and emergencies—they should have a written plan. Also, make sure they have a copy of your emergency plan. Among the questions to ask:

- How will they contact me if it's an emergency?
- Whom can they contact if I am not available?
- If the center or school has to be evacuated, where do they go?
- What kind of emergency supplies do they have on hand? For how many children and how many days?

your child's backpack and in the glove compartment of your car. Also make sure all caregivers—including the babysitter—have a copy.

The plan should include:

- **Emergency meeting locations.** You need two: a specific place outside your home such as a curbside mailbox or a neighbor's driveway to gather in the event of a household emergency such as a fire; and another location outside your neighborhood like the local school in case you can't return home during a local or regional disaster.
  If you have Internet access after a regional disaster, you also can register on the Red Cross's Safe and Well List at *www.redcross.org* to report your status or search for a loved one. You should also become familiar with your child's daycare or school disaster plans in case you're separated during an emergency (see tip box, this page, and page 26), and make sure you are familiar with any disaster plans at your workplace.

- **Emergency phone number.** This should be a local phone number for family members to call in the event of an emergency. It is important that everyone in your family, including your children, know to call this number as soon as they are safe. It might be your cell phone or the phone number of a friend or neighbor.
- **An out-of-town contact person.** Ask a relative or friend who lives outside your area to be your emergency contact person. After a disaster, it is often easier to make a long-distance call than a local call from the impacted area because telephones lines may be down or jammed.
- **A family communication plan.** This is a list of important phone numbers and Web sites. It should include telephone, cell phone and e-mail contact information for all family members, work, school and your out-of-town emergency person. Also include meeting locations, community emergency services contact information and information for the National Poison Control Center hotline (800-222-1222).

You can find a sample form for recording this information in Chapter 6: Family Resources or at *www.ready.gov* or *www.redcross.org/contactcard*. Make a copy for everyone to keep with them. Also, post the list by your home telephone, keep one in the glove compartment of your vehicle and one in your desk or locker at work. Also teach your children how to call the contact numbers and when it is appropriate to do so.

Escape Plans and Safe Places
You may have to evacuate at a moment's notice, so be ready to get out *fast*. Make sure everyone in your family knows the best escape routes out of the home and out of the area and make sure you have more than one option.

This is why it's so important to keep a regional map with an emergency preparedness kit. Mark your evacuation routes on the map and drive them in

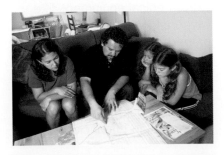

advance to become familiar with the routes. If you don't drive or own a motor vehicle, find out what arrangements local officials have made for evacuating those without private transportation.

Practice both your home and area evacuation drills at least twice a year and whenever you update your escape plan. However, in the event of an emergency, always listen to the television or radio and take the emergency routes officials recommend.

Plan for Family Members with Disabilities and Medical Needs. Make sure your emergency plan includes plans for someone with disabilities. If your child is blind, deaf or in a wheelchair, how will he or she get out of the home or region?

Also, make sure you include a copy of medical records, medication prescriptions, a 3-day supply of medications and extra medical equipment, like oxygen, in your emergency preparedness kit. You should also give the power company a list of any power-dependent life-support equipment your family member requires and develop a back-up plan that includes an alternate power source for the equipment or for relocating the person if the power goes out.

Don't forget to complete an Emergency Information Form for each child with medical health needs. You can find one at *www.aap.org/ advocacy/emergprep.htm.*

Include Your Pets. If you must evacuate, take your pets with you. If it's not safe for you, it's not safe for them. But be aware that the Red Cross and other public emergency shelters often do not accept pets (except service animals) because of sanitation reasons. So prepare a list of family, friends, boarding facilities, veterinarians and pet-friendly motels/hotels that can shelter your pets in an emergency.

Be Informed

It's important to learn about the types of disasters that could happen where you live and the appropriate response to those situations. Do you live in an area that is prone to flash floods or tornadoes? Is your community in a hurricane or earthquake hazard area?

Your local emergency management office can inform

you about how authorities will warn of a pending disaster and provide information during and afterward. During a disaster, listen to your battery-powered radio to stay informed about evacuation routes, emergency shelters, food and water distribution centers and other crucial information.

A good information source is the NOAA Weather Radio (NWR), a nationwide network of radio stations that broadcasts National Weather Service warnings, watches, forecasts and other hazard information 24 hours a day. NWR also broadcasts warning and post-event information for other hazards, including natural (earthquakes or avalanches), environmental (chemical releases or oil spills) and public safety (AMBER alerts or 9-1-1 telephone outages). To access NWR broadcasts you need a special radio or scanner capable of picking up the signal. For more information, visit *www.nws.noaa.gov* and click on Weather Radio.

Learn First Aid/CPR

Seconds count during a medical emergency. There won't be time to look up information in a book. That's why it's crucial that you,

other adults and older children in your family know what to do for various types of medical emergencies now. Review the first aid and CPR information in Chapter 3: Life-Threatening First Aid Emergencies (see page 51) as soon as possible to be prepared for a medical emergency.

While this information is a good start, it is not intended as a substitute for the training and materials you can receive in a Red Cross First Aid and CPR certification course. Contact your local Red Cross chapter to sign up for a training class today. Then, persuade at least one other member of your family to go with you for training. Your family's safety is well worth this small investment of your time.

Share What You Learned

Neighbors can help each other save lives and property by working together during a disaster. Share what you've learned about emergency preparedness with your neighbors now, before an emergency occurs, and discuss how everyone in the neighborhood can help one another during and after a disaster.

If you belong to a neighborhood organization, such as a homeowners' association or a community crime watch group, develop a presentation on disaster preparedness.

Also identify neighbors with special medical and technical skills and think about how you can assist those with special needs, such as the disabled and elderly.

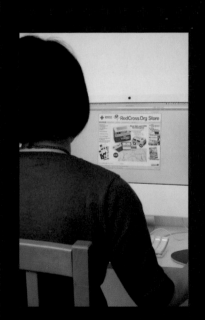

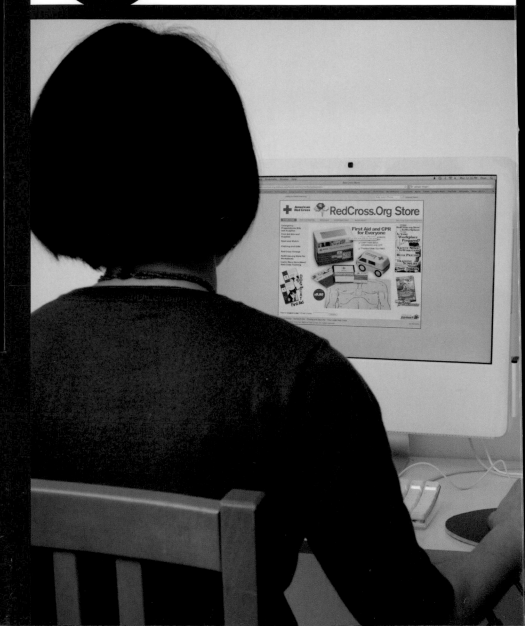

Family Resources

As a parent, it is important to know how to provide first aid, prevent your child from being injured and respond during an emergency. Check out the following resources for more information.

Web Sites and Other Information Resources

American Red Cross
- Web site: *www.redcross.org*
- Enter your zip code at "Find" to locate your local American Red Cross chapter. Click on "Get Prepared" to learn how to be prepared for disasters at home, school and at work. From "Prepare at School," click the link to "Masters of Disaster" to download children's activities, drawings and puzzle sheets.
- Visit *www.redcross.org/beredcrossready* for a free online education module on how to "get a kit", "make a plan" and "be informed" about emergency preparedness.

American Academy of Pediatrics
- Web site: *www.aap.org*
- Excellent source of information on keeping your children safe and healthy from the nation's premier organization of pediatricians.

American Association of Poison Control Centers
- Web site: *www.aapcc.org*
- Click on "Poison Prevention and Education" as well as "Games" to learn how to prevent poisoning accidents.
- **Hotline: 800-222-1222 (call this number for a poisoning emergency)**

Centers for Disease Control and Prevention
- Web site: *www.cdc.gov*
- Learn about disease processes and prevention.

Citizen Corps
- Web site: *www.CitizenCorps.gov*
- Learn how to get involved in your local Citizen Corps Council and make a difference in your community.

Consumer Product Safety Commission
- Web site: *www.cpsc.gov*
- Learn about product safety standards and recalls.

Federal Emergency Management Agency
- Web site: *www.fema.gov*
- Learn about regional disasters and other emergencies that have impacted your area and how to be better prepared for them.

Kids Health
- Web site: *www.KidsHealth.org*
- Provides doctor-approved health information about children from before birth through adolescence.

National Fire Protection Association
- Web site: *www.nfpa.org*
- A wealth of fire and burn prevention information, including kids pages and activities featuring "Sparky" the dog.

Poison Prevention
- Web site: *www.poisonprevention.org*
- Provides information about the events associated with National Poison Prevention Week, the steps that you can take to help prevent accidental poisonings and tips for promoting community involvement in poison prevention.

Safe Kids Worldwide
- Web site: *www.usa.safekids.org*
- Excellent source of safety information for parents.

American Red Cross
Emergency Contact Card

Directions:

1. Make a copy of this card for each family member.
2. Cut out the card along the dotted lines.
3. Write contact information of those who should be called in the event of an emergency, including home, work and mobile phone numbers.
4. After discussing with other family members, also write down your out-of-area contact person and where your family will gather in the event of a regional disaster. (For more information on how to create a family disaster plan and assemble an emergency supplies kit, as well as other valuable preparedness information, review Chapter 5, pages 105-116, and visit *www.redcross.org*.)
5. On the back of the card, list current medical conditions and medications, both prescription and over-the-counter.
6. Fold the card so it fits in your pocket, wallet or purse.
7. Have each family member carry this card on their person at all times so you—or emergency medical responders—will have quick access to vital information if it is needed.

Visit **www.redcross.org** for more information.

Family Doctor:

Poison Control Center: 800-222-1222

Ambulance: Call 9-1-1 or

Police: Call 9-1-1 or

Fire Dept.: Call 9-1-1 or

Important Phone Numbers

Emergency Contact Card

American Red Cross

Name:

Home Address:

Phone Number:

Family Members Contact Information

Doctor:

Out-of-town contact:

Family meeting place outside the neighborhood:

Medical Conditions

FOLD—

FOLD—

Medications

☐ Rx
☐ OTC

☐ Rx
☐ OTC

☐ Rx
☐ OTC

☐ Rx
☐ OTC

☐ Rx
☐ OTC

FOLD—
☐ Rx
☐ OTC

☐ Rx
☐ OTC

☐ Rx
☐ OTC

☐ Rx
☐ OTC

☐ Rx
☐ OTC

Prevent Injuries, Avoid Illnesses and Keep Your Family Safe...You Can Do It!

With the American Red Cross Safety Series, Everything You Need Is at Your Fingertips.

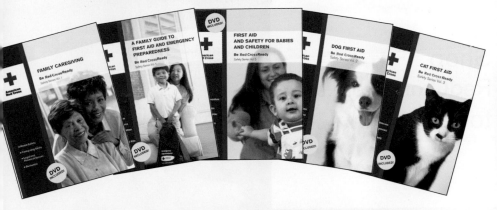

Helping Your Family and Your Community Stay Safe Just Got Easier.

The American Red Cross Safety Series makes it easy to help your family, friends and neighbors stay safe. These easy-to-read guides are designed to help you find information quickly in the event of an emergency. Each one features full color photos and a DVD that helps you and your family build skills even faster. Plus, the guides were developed by the Red Cross, in consultation with leading experts, so you know this is information you can trust.

The Red Cross Safety Series includes these important topics:
• Family Caregiving
• A Family Guide to First Aid and Emergency Preparedness
• First Aid and Safety for Babies and Children
• Dog First Aid
• Cat First Aid

Complete Your Safety Series Today– Visit www.redcross.org/store.

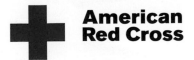

Keep your peace of mind close at hand.

Shop RedCrossStore.org today.

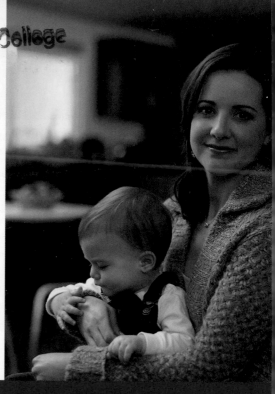

Visit RedCrossStore.org today to purchase first aid and emergency preparedness kits to store at home, work and in the car. Check out our free **Be Red Cross Ready** interactive presentation to learn more about important steps you can take to prepare your family for emergencies.

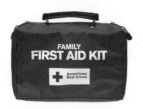

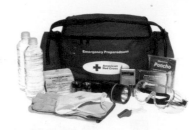

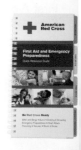

Be Red Cross Ready

American Red Cross